SCRAMBLING FOR AFRICA

EXPERTISE

**CULTURES AND
TECHNOLOGIES
OF KNOWLEDGE**

EDITED BY DOMINIC BOYER

A list of titles in this series is available at www.cornellpress.cornell.edu

SCRAMBLING FOR AFRICA

AIDS, Expertise, and the Rise of American Global Health Science

JOHANNA TAYLOE CRANE

CORNELL UNIVERSITY PRESS
ITHACA AND LONDON

First published 2013 by Cornell University Press
First printing, Cornell Paperbacks, 2013
Printed in the United States of America

Library of Congress Cataloging-in-Publication Data

Crane, Johanna Tayloe, author.
    Scrambling for Africa : AIDS, Expertise, and the rise of American
global health science / Johanna Tayloe Crane.
        pages cm
    Includes bibliographical references and index.
    ISBN 978-0-8014-5195-9 (cloth : alk. paper)
    ISBN 978-0-8014-7917-5 (pbk : alk. paper)
    1. Medical anthropology–Uganda.   2. AIDS (Disease)–Research–
Uganda.   3. Medical assistance, American–Uganda.   I. Title.

    GN296.5.U33C73 2013
    306.4'61096761–dc23   2013001257

Cornell University Press strives to use environmentally responsible
suppliers and materials to the fullest extent possible in the publishing of
its books. Such materials include vegetable-based, low-VOC inks and
acid-free papers that are recycled, totally chlorine-free, or partly composed
of nonwood fibers. For further information visit our website at www
.cornellpress.cornell.edu.

Cloth printing   10   9   8   7   6   5   4   3   2   1
Paperback printing   10   9   8   7   6   5   4   3   2   1

For my mother and father

"The negotiation on the equivalence of nonequivalent situations
is always what characterizes the spread of a science."
BRUNO LATOUR, 1983

Contents

Acknowledgments

This book is the product of nearly a decade of work, and I have many people to thank for bringing it to fruition. My first debt goes to the researchers and doctors who appear under pseudonyms in these pages, especially Jason Beale, whose remarkable openness and professional generosity made this ethnography possible, both by allowing me access to his research process and by connecting me with many of the researchers and doctors interviewed for this book. Special thanks also go to Dr. John Atuhaire, who provided me with several lengthy interviews over the years and assisted me with the IRB application process at the Mbarara University of Science and Technology, and Eve Ozobia, who helped with contacts on the ground in Mbarara and also provided some of the sharpest and most nuanced insights into the social relations of transnational research. I also thank Dr. Willa Balozi for welcoming my presence at the Immune Wellness Clinic, helping arrange interviews with clinic doctors, and for allowing me to observe staff meetings. And although she appears only briefly in these pages, my deepest gratitude goes to Idah Mukyala, whose friendship, support, and kind heart sustained me during my trips to Uganda and who assisted me with this project in innumerable ways. *Mukama akukume bulungi.*

This work originated nearly ten years ago as my dissertation research in the University of California, San Francisco–University of California, Berkeley Joint Program in Medical Anthropology. As a graduate student, my research and writing was supported by grants and fellowships from the Human Rights Center at UC Berkeley, the Philanthropic Educational Organization, the Institute for Health Policy Studies at UCSF, the University of California Universitywide AIDS Research Program, the National Science Foundation Science and Technology Studies Program, and the University of California Humanities Research Institute. The faculty and my fellow graduate students in the UCSF Department of Anthropology, History, and Social Medicine and the UC Berkeley Department of Anthropology created a fertile intellectual environment for work at the intersections of critical medical anthropology and science studies during the time I was there, which undoubtedly shaped the trajectory of my research. I am particularly grateful to Cori Hayden and Warwick Anderson for their guidance, to Vincanne Adams for her ongoing mentorship and enthusiasm, and to Philippe Bourgois for his support and encouragement since I first studied under him at San Francisco State University. It was through working closely with Philippe and Vincanne that I realized I could do an ethnography of science that was also about power and inequality. I also wish to credit Donald Moore for introducing me to the fruitful connections between cultural geography and anthropology during my time as a graduate student.

I was supported during the long project of working on this book by Mellon postdoctoral fellowships at Cornell University's Department of Science and Technology Studies and the University of Pennsylvania Penn Humanities Forum, and by a Stetten Fellowship from the Office of History at the National Institutes of Health (NIH). I thank the faculty and students in the Cornell Science and Technology Studies department, especially Michael Lynch, Trevor Pinch, Stephen Hilgartner, Suman Seth, Rachel Prentice, Kathleen Vogel, Sarah Pritchard, Jessica Ratcliff, and Manjari Mahajan for their interest in my project and their feedback on work that eventually made it into some of the chapters included here. I also thank the Cornell Society for the Humanities for awarding a Mellon Grant for an Interdisciplinary Writing Group on "Centering Africa" to myself and six colleagues, which allowed me to further develop my project in the excellent company of Dan

Magaziner, Stacey Langwick, Dagmawi Woubshet, Sandra Greene, Judith Byfield, and Jeremy Foster, all of whom helped attune me to important perspectives and themes in African Studies. At the University of Pennsylvania, my proposal for this book and early chapter drafts benefitted from the input of colleagues at the Penn Humanities Forum seminar on "Connections," and especially from my fellow Forum fellows, Jennifer Borland, Sindhu Revuluri, Chiara Cilleri, and Andrew Witmer. I am also grateful for conversations with faculty and graduate students in the Department of History and Sociology of Science at the University of Pennsylvania, especially Steven Feierman, Robbie Aronowitz, Marissa Mika, and Erica Dwyer.

When it comes to writing, I have never been very good at multitasking. For this reason, I am indebted to the NIH Office of History, where a Stetten Fellowship allowed me a year without teaching during which I was able to draft the bulk of this manuscript. My colleagues there, especially Robert Martensen, David Cantor, Sejal Patel, and Marian Moser Jones, provided valuable feedback and constructive criticism on first drafts of chapters 3 and 4. I also wish to acknowledge the National Institutes of Allergy and Infectious Disease for providing financial support for my Stetten Fellowship.

A short-term fellowship from the Chemical Heritage Foundation supported me during the summer of 2009, and during the summer of 2010, I was fortunate enough to be a guest of the research group on the anthropology of Law, Organization, Science, and Technology (LOST) at the Max Planck Institute for Social Anthropology in Halle, Germany. I thank Richard Rottenburg for this opportunity, and for including me in the LOST group's 2010 Conference on Bodies and Bodiliness in Africa, where I circulated a first draft of chapter 5. I have Richard and the participants in that conference to thank for helping me recognize the value of a careful critique, rather than a blunt condemnation, of the social relations of global health science.

Since arriving at the University of Washington–Bothell in 2011, I have been nurtured by the campus's collegial environment, inquisitive students, and the unique interdisciplinary intellectual community that exists at the School of Interdisciplinary Arts and Sciences. I am particularly grateful to the members of my cross-campus writing group—Ron Krabill, Ben Gardner, Lynn Thomas, and Danny Hoffman—for providing me with much-needed feedback on the introduction, chapter 1, and conclusion to this book.

It has been a pleasure and an honor to work with Cornell University Press. I thank Peter Potter for his support and guidance throughout the writing and editorial process, and Dominic Boyer for his responsiveness, insightful editorial suggestions, and ready willingness to read revised chapter drafts along the way. I am also grateful to the manuscript's two anonymous reviewers, who gave helpful advice about how to address certain gaps and inconsistencies in the text, and whose positive responses to the manuscript buoyed my spirits. In addition to the anonymous reviewers, Dan Magaziner, Julie Livingston, Suman Seth, and Marissa Mika deserve special mention for their willingness to read a draft of the full manuscript. I am grateful to all of them for their generosity, and especially to Dan, who took the time to sit and discuss the draft with me for several hours over his dining room table, and Julie, who sent me extensive written comments along with one of the kindest emails I have ever received regarding my work. Their feedback was invaluable. Any remaining shortcomings or errors within the text are, of course, exclusively my own.

Two of the chapters included in this book have been previously published in somewhat altered forms as journal articles. An earlier version of chapter 2 was published in 2011 in *BioSocieties* under the title, "Viral Cartographies." Parts of chapter 5 appeared in 2010 as an article entitled "Unequal Partners" in *Behemoth: A Journal on Civilization*.

Although research and writing requires financial and intellectual support, it also requires emotional support. Over the past decade I have made homes in five different cities, seven different apartments, and four states. I survived, and even thrived, during this time of transience because I am blessed with a community of friends and family whose love and loyalty I value more than anything else in this world. Here I name just a few whose actions made this book possible. Paula Zenti first took me into the residence hotels of San Francisco. Emily Lewis offered support, encouragement, and humor via lengthy emails during my trips to Uganda. Alexandra Choby kept me company during the long and often lonely process of dissertation writing. Hillary Brooks provided a welcoming and happy home in Oakland at a time when I needed it most. Becka Warren's friendship and loyalty sustained me over the ups and downs of most of my adult life, and continues to do so. I am honored to be "fictive kin" to her, Jason, Clementine, and Max.

Lastly, my most profound gratitude belongs to my family. My brother Lee, sister-in-law Mina, and my aunt Pam provided warm and welcome company and beds to sleep in when I was commuting between Philadelphia and Bethesda. Kristian Boose has provided steadfast emotional support, loving companionship, and much-needed study breaks throughout the process of completing this manuscript. I am grateful every day for his generous heart, his curiosity, and his kind spirit. Most of all I am thankful to my parents, Dorothy and Dod Crane, who taught me to be inquisitive, open-minded, loyal, and fair, and whose unwavering love has anchored me throughout my life. This book is dedicated to them.

Scrambling for Africa

INTRODUCTION

My first visit to Mbarara's Immune Wellness Clinic[1] was in July of 2003, when I spent a day there as part of a visiting research team from San Francisco, California. Located about four hours south of Kampala, Uganda's capital city, the town of Mbarara is surrounded by rolling grassy hills that turn golden in the dry season. It is cattle and dairy country, and the main streets of the town center are dotted with shops selling fresh local milk by the ladle-full. The Wellness Clinic is located at the edge of town, on the grounds of the university teaching hospital with which it is affiliated. We arrived at the collection of low-lying cement buildings that make up the

---

1. The name of the clinic is a pseudonym, but all other place names used in the book are real unless otherwise noted. All individuals named in this ethnography are referred to using pseudonyms in order to protect privacy. The exceptions to this are when I refer to individuals quoted in public forums, such as the press or scientific conferences, in which case I use real names. On rare occasions, I have combined two individuals into a single composite character in order to stream-line the manuscript and make the number of names more manageable for the reader.

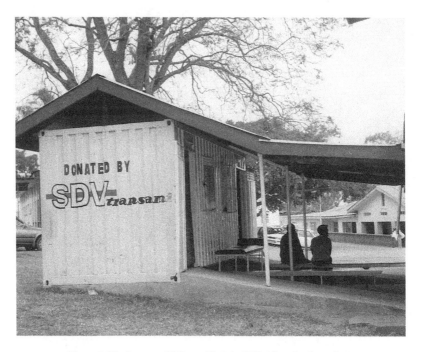

Figure 1: The Immune Wellness Clinic in 2003 (photo by the author).

hospital at about 10:30 that morning. When we asked around for the office of Dr. Harry Salter, the American missionary who had founded the clinic, someone instructed us to walk up the hill to the "containers." Initially puzzled by these instructions, we soon learned that the clinic was housed in a donated metal shipping container—the same kind we were accustomed to seeing at home, in our peripheral vision, as we passed the Oakland shipyards when crossing the San Francisco Bay. The container-clinic was divided into two small exam rooms, each with a doorway covered by a cloth curtain. At the time, it was the only dedicated HIV clinic in all of southwestern Uganda.

One of the patients we met on that day in 2003 was a friendly and helpful man named Gabriel Muzoora. Gabriel was a widower caring for three children. No longer able to work as a carpenter due to his poor health, he supported himself on the small stipend he earned drumming in a song and dance group affiliated with The AIDS Support Organization (TASO), Uganda's best-known HIV education and support organization. He regularly made the 20-kilometer trip between his rural home and the Wellness Clinic via minibus taxi (one of the principal means of shared transit in Uganda), even though his inability to afford the anti-HIV (antiretroviral) medications sold at the clinic's pharmacy meant that the care he received there could do little to forestall the disease's inevitable progression.

Dr. Salter had opened the clinic in 1997 under the auspices of the Faculty of Medicine at Mbarara University of Science and Technology (MUST), where he held a teaching position. With support from his Baptist missionary organization, the clinic was able to provide what Ugandans would call "small drugs," such as antibiotics, for free. However, it had no means of subsidizing the very effective but expensive multidrug antiretroviral "cocktails" that were by then the standard of care for AIDS patients in the United States. The discovery of these drugs in 1995 and their seemingly miraculous ability to restore health to patients near death is often heralded as the dawn of the AIDS "treatment era." Yet, in Uganda and most other low-income countries, this breakthrough initially had very little impact, since the high price of the medications—easily US$15,000 yearly—kept them out of reach to all but the wealthy. Globally, activists and advocates fought for humanitarian aid and drug pricing policies that would support free access to the treatments in poor countries, especially in sub-Saharan Africa, where two-thirds of the world's people with AIDS resided (UNAIDS and WHO 2006). But international donors hesitated, arguing that impoverished patients might take the medicines improperly and generate dangerous strains of drug-resistant virus. Things began to shift in 2001, when generic drug manufacturers in India and elsewhere began manufacturing and exporting cheaper "copycat" antiretroviral combinations to African countries. By 2003 these Indian drugs were available for just under US$30 a month at a handful of clinic pharmacies in Uganda (including the Wellness Clinic), but in a country where over half the population earned under $1.25 a day, this price remained unaffordable for Gabriel and many other people living with AIDS (UNDP 2010). As a result, for the first decade of the "treatment era," most people with AIDS in Uganda and other low-income countries were dying no differently than they had in the 1980s.

Only a few years later, the situation had changed radically. Through pressure from treatment activists and a growing concern that the epidemic might cause political instability in the region, the United States and other wealthy nations came to frame AIDS in Africa as an emergency in need of direct humanitarian action. This political shift, in combination with falling drug prices, ushered in the establishment of the multinational Global Fund to Fight AIDS, Tuberculosis, and Malaria and the U.S. President's Emergency Plan for AIDS Relief (PEPFAR) in the early 2000s. These two major, internationally financed HIV-treatment programs reshaped the landscape of global HIV treatment access by providing significant financial support for free antiretroviral treatment in poor countries. By late 2004, these programs had begun to supply clinics across Africa with free antiretrovirals and other drugs and services for HIV patients. Health policy discussions shifted away from debates over whether or not African patients could take antiretrovirals properly and refocused on concerns over clinic and laboratory infrastructure, staffing shortages, and the long-term sustainability of foreign-funded treatment programs. Although treatment access today remains far from universal, there is no doubt that these programs have profoundly impacted the lives of AIDS patients, their families, and their care providers in recipient nations. As of May 2009, over 5,000 individuals—including Gabriel—were being treated with free HIV medications in Mbarara.

The first decade of the new millennium also brought other big changes to the Wellness Clinic. Although the advent of free antiretrovirals was certainly the most important shift in terms of human survival, the influx of international funding also fueled the rapid growth of AIDS-related infrastructure and research on the adjacent medical school campus. Indeed, a visitor to the clinic in 2009 would be hard pressed to find the original "container" clinic, as it had been absorbed into an ever-growing complex of new buildings crowding the northeastern corner of the hospital grounds. Largely financed by PEPFAR and other American partners, these buildings were used to provide much-needed space for the HIV clinic's growing staff of clinicians and counselors, as well as new laboratory and pharmacy services. In addition, they accommodated a rapidly expanding and largely U.S.-funded scientific apparatus focused on studying the rollout of antiretroviral treatment in Africa and the impact of the powerful drugs on thousands of never-before-treated patients. Such a biological "blank slate" was unavailable in wealthy countries, where antiretrovirals had been readily available for nearly a decade.

At the vanguard of this influx of foreign researchers to Mbarara was Dr. Jason Beale, a physician-researcher who had begun his clinical career as an AIDS doctor in New York City and San Francisco in the 1980s, working on the front lines of the American HIV epidemic in the years before effective antiretrovirals. Dr. Beale first came to Uganda in the early 2000s, in search of a location for a new research study examining antiretroviral access, medication adherence, and HIV drug resistance in Africa. He knew that the availability of antiretrovirals (ARVs) was on the rise and that international funding for treatment was likely to come soon, and he was hoping to find a clinic where he could study patients as they received the drugs for the first time. While spending time in Kampala, he met Dr. John Atuhaire, a young medical officer from the Immune Wellness Clinic in Mbarara, who was visiting the capital to attend a training program designed to teach African doctors about how to care for patients on antiretroviral treatment. Atuhaire had brought with him a handwritten register where he had been recording basic information about the clinic's growing number of patients purchasing generic, Indian-manufactured antiretroviral therapy. As he showed Beale the register, Atuhaire explained that as more and more patients were able to access ARVs, it was becoming increasingly difficult for him—the clinic's only full-time doctor—to keep the records current.

Beale saw valuable data in Atuhaire's register—and an opportunity for collaboration. Mbarara's hospital and medical school were largely off the beaten track for international researchers, who tended to work in and around the capital city. Beale was one of the first foreigners to propose a research partnership, and when he visited the Mbarara University of Science and Technology, he found the faculty eager for opportunities to collaborate. He quickly forged an agreement with Dr. Atuhaire and Dr. Salter to develop a pilot study of the Immune Wellness Clinic's patients, and to provide the clinic with an electronic record-keeping system. In a fitting symmetry, Beale's pilot research project would also be housed in a shipping container on the hospital's grounds, as this was the only available space at the time. The container was empty and abandoned, but Dr. Salter offered it to him on the condition that Beale pay for the necessary renovations (a cost of about $100) and reserve half of the container for additional clinic rooms. In the United States, Beale was accustomed to grappling with substantial academic and government bureaucracies in order to secure research space, and he was pleasantly surprised by the ease with which he was able to acquire a spot in Mbarara. As he described it, the whole arrangement was negotiated over a twenty-minute conversation ending with a handshake. Two weeks later, the container was renovated and ready for use.

From these modest beginnings, Beale's research endeavor would grow into a multistudy, multi-institution operation by the end of the decade. When I visited in 2009, I counted nearly twenty ongoing or recently completed research projects funded by Beale's grants or those of his American collaborators, and I learned that the studies now employed over seventy people in Mbarara. This sizeable international research presence, combined with the substantial influx of funds, staffing, and infrastructure via PEPFAR, meant that when Gabriel and other HIV patients attended their doctors' appointments in 2009, they encountered a clinic that had been transformed since its earlier days. Instead of awaiting their appointments outdoors in front of the container clinic, patients sat inside a new two-story clinic building on benches outside the doctors' offices. In addition to doctors and nurses, a small army of laboratory and data entry personnel made their way up and down the clinic hallways, joined occasionally by visiting researchers from Baltimore, Boston, or San Francisco. When examining patients, doctors no longer took visit notes in longhand, but instead recorded relevant clinical findings on a "patient encounter form" that had been standardized with a series of checkboxes to facilitate data entry. These records, as well as laboratory reports documenting a patient's CD4 (T cell) count and viral load results, were kept in the clinic's designated "data room," where data entry staff typed their contents into an American-designed Excel database on a bank of nine desktop computers. In short, Gabriel and the thousands of other HIV-positive Ugandans registered at the clinic were no longer simply targets of care, but also fodder for the generation of scientific knowledge.

Inequality and the Making of Global Health Science

The story of the Immune Wellness Clinic is a telling one. In the space of a decade, Africa went from a continent largely excluded from advancements in HIV medicine to an area of central concern and knowledge production within the increasingly popular field of "global health science." As I chronicle in chapter 1, in the early 2000s, African countries were dismissed as too poor and chaotic to benefit from the high-tech antiretroviral medications that had transformed HIV care and life expectancies in the United States and Europe. Western experts argued that Africa risked becoming a place of "antiretroviral anarchy" and a "'petri dish' for new treatment-resistant strains" (Harries et al. 2001; Popp and Fisher 2002). A decade later, as I write this, Uganda and other African nations find themselves courted by some of the most prestigious research universities in the world as they scramble to find "resource-poor" hospitals in which to base their international HIV research and global health programs. Notably, many of these institutions are U.S. universities, which have seen an explosion of interest and investment in "global health" research and education since the turn of the millennium (Merson and Page 2009). "Africa," as Dr. Beale told me in 2005, "is in vogue now."

This transformation, while crucial for new arrangements in the provision of care and the production of knowledge, is far from neutral. Using Uganda and the United States as linked sites, this book rests on the premise that AIDS in Africa has been not only a source of tragic misfortune and death, but also fodder for profound institutional and intellectual opportunity. However, these opportunities are meted out unevenly, and have produced fresh inequalities. I argue that one outcome of this uncomfortable mix of preventable suffering and scientific productivity has been the making of a "global health science" that paradoxically embodies and even benefits from the very inequalities it aspires to redress. Within global health, the very characteristics that once led some Western experts to dismiss HIV treatment in Africa as unwise—impoverished patients, poor infrastructure, understaffed health facilities—are now those that make many African countries attractive as "resource-poor settings" that can offer "global" research and educational opportunities unavailable in "resource-rich settings" like the United States. In other words, to global health, these are *valuable inequalities*. This is true not only for American experts and institutions, but also for their African collaborators, who—like Dr. Salter and Dr. Atuhaire—may find that their ability to grant (or foreclose) access to their patients serves as a form of currency in a transnational research economy fueled by data.

This book is an ethnographic examination of the ways in which global health science both generates and relies upon inequalities, even as it strives to end them. I examine this paradox across a series of interlinked scales, ranging from the molecular tools used to study and treat HIV to the transnational funding apparatuses that underwrite global health research. My intent is to offer a critical geography of expertise that provincializes the

"Western" AIDS science that is often accepted as universal and challenges the historical placement of Africa and Africans at the periphery of scientific knowledge making (Chakrabarty 2000). One element of this critical geography entails tracking the effects of the complex interplay between science, technology, and global inequality in modest, up-country African clinics like the one I describe in Mbarara. But it also necessitates turning an ethnographic eye toward the production of knowledge in laboratories and conference rooms in wealthy American cities like San Francisco and Seattle, and examining the processes by which our often taken-for-granted tools of knowledge making, such as surveys, databases, and laboratory assays, are built, and what they include and exclude.

Because of its close kinship to medical humanitarianism, global health science can be challenging to critique (Fassin 2010a). Both fields share a moral commitment to "saving lives," and it can feel petty to criticize the approaches of scientists and others striving to improve health in impoverished parts of the world. Given the initial sluggishness of the Western response to HIV/AIDS in Africa, the current enthusiasm for studying and ameliorating global health inequalities is a welcome shift. But good intentions and compassionate action are not immune to the power imbalances and inequalities they seek to redress, and it is thus crucial that we do not obviate critical thinking about that which is done "in the name of global health" (MacFarlane, Jacobs, and Kaaya 2008). Global health, like humanitarianism, is not only a moral endeavor aimed at assisting victims of disease, but also "a political resource (serving specific interests) to justify action considered to be in favor of others exposed to a vital danger, action taken in the name of a shared humanity" (Fassin 2010b, 239; Redfield 2005; Redfield and Bornstein 2010). For this reason, we must seek empirical answers to the questions who is global health science for? Who benefits, and how? What new "species of biocapital" are forged when poverty and inequality are invoked as both the enemy and, paradoxically, the fuel of global health (Helmreich 2008)?

Addressing these questions necessitates critical ethnographic attention to the connections between two kinds of places, often dichotomized as American and African, "industrialized" and "developing," donor nation and aid recipient, global North and global South. This dichotomization, while certainly valid in many respects, is nonetheless misleading in its emphasis on that which differentiates and divides these places, rather than the many ways in which they are entangled. In contrast, this ethnography brings together seemingly disjunctive entities: American university doctors and Ugandan lab technicians, crack users in San Francisco and AIDS experts in Kampala, French viruses and Indian pharmaceutical companies, the U.S. National Institutes of Health and Ugandan university administrators, the practice of science and the legacy of colonialism, the epidemiologist and the anthropologist. It is through exploring this mosaic, this "global assemblage" (Ong and Collier 2005), that the politics of global health science become palpable and available for critical analysis.

Biomedical Expertise in Postcolonial Uganda

In the introduction to her excellent ethnography of medical training in Malawi, Claire Wendland outlines the "two stories of biomedicine abroad" most often recounted in the academic literature: biomedicine as a humanitarian, altruistic endeavor, and biomedicine as a hegemonic tool of domination over indigenous knowledge. In both stories, biomedicine is figured as an "essentially Western" field that is exported elsewhere (Wendland 2010, 14). Such a formulation leaves little space for the consideration of African biomedical expertise and practice. (I should note here that this book focuses fairly narrowly on the practices of biomedical experts in contemporary Uganda and the United States. There is a large literature on health and healing in Africa that covers many important issues not examined in this ethnography, including the social nature of illness and medicine in Africa, indigenous and "traditional" medical practices and epistemologies, colonial and missionary medicine, and the experiences of sufferers and families. See, for example, Janzen 1982; Packard 1989; Vaughan 1991; Feierman and Janzen 1992; Hunt 1999; Thomas 2003; Bledsoe 2002; Livingston 2005, 2012; Luedke and West 2006; Foley 2010; Langwick 2011).

Ugandans have been practicing professional biomedicine for nearly as long as Americans have. In the United States, the biomedical profession in its modern form arose following the publication of the Flexner Report in 1910. This report called for the standardization of medical education curricula and the elimination of "proprietary" non-college-affiliated medical trade schools, thus bringing U.S. medical education more in line with European practices and standards (Starr 1982). It was during this same time period that biomedicine also began to emerge as a profession within

Uganda, first through classes offered at the Mengo missionary hospital in 1917, but principally through the initiation of medical training at Makerere University in 1923. Established in Kampala under British colonial rule, Makerere's medical school was intended to train Ugandans and other East Africans to become local providers of biomedical care as "senior native (later African) medical assistants." Although training was similar to that offered in Britain, graduates were not allowed to call themselves "doctors" and were licensed to practice medicine only in government service. Seeking professional legitimacy and the ability to establish private practices, Makerere graduates fought to have their medical degrees recognized by Britain's General Medical Council during the 1940s and 50s (Iliffe 2002). They eventually succeeded, and recognition was granted in 1957. Five years later, Uganda became an independent nation.

The 1960s are generally regarded as the heyday of Ugandan biomedicine, as Makerere Medical School (along with its teaching hospital, Mulago) "became a research and teaching center of international reputation" (Iliffe 2002, 140). Research flourished, buoyed by an influx of foreign funding, and Ugandan and expatriate scientists produced important findings both on disease patterns within East Africa and on so-called "Western" ailments such as cancer and heart disease. Ugandan cancer research, in particular, was considered to be of "major international importance" in its suggestion of links between certain cancers and viral infections (ibid., 142–3; Mika 2009; Livingston 2012). This era of productivity came to an abrupt and violent end under the military dictatorship of General Idi Amin (1971 to 1979), when, as members of the elite, Ugandan doctors and medical school professors became targets of violence and killing, leading many to flee the country. Relative stability returned with the takeover of Yoweri Museveni in 1986, but the government health sector—including the medical school and Mulago teaching hospital—was left weak, underfunded, and largely dependent upon foreign aid (Dodge and Wiebe 1985; Allen 1991; Bond and Vincent 1991; Whyte 1991).

Nonetheless, Uganda's history as a premier place for biomedical education and research in East Africa left it with a core of highly trained medical experts, even after years of political turmoil and economic decline. It was these researchers, in collaboration with American and British colleagues, who would publish some of the first scientific papers on clinical and epidemiological aspects of AIDS in Africa. This work made critical contributions to scientific understandings of the new disease, especially its hetero-sexual transmission and association with Kaposi's sarcoma and tuberculosis (Serwadda et al. 1985; Sewankambo et al. 1987a, 1987b; Nambuya et al. 1988; Katongole-Mbidde, Banura, and Nakakeeto 1989). Many of these physician-scientists remain notable figures among Uganda's scientific elite. Based in Kampala, they often hold prominent positions at Makerere and have sig-nificant ties to foreign universities and international funding bodies, which seek them out as collaborators or "partners" in global health research endeav-ors. In turn, aspiring researchers in outlying towns (such as Mbarara) may cultivate relationships with these senior colleagues in Kampala in an effort to gain access to the transnational scientific networks in which the capital city is a key nodal point.

Ugandan doctors and researchers both embrace and chafe against the foreign programs and institutions that simultaneously enable and constrain their work. This ambivalent relationship bears some echoes of the colonial era, when East African doctors relied upon the British state for medical training and employment even as they struggled with it over professional recognition and equality. This relationship between doctors and the colo-nial state, rather than being one of overt conflict, was one of "uneasy sym-biosis" (Iliffe 2002, 4). In the current postcolonial era, the role formerly played by the colonizing state is now partly filled by "donors": the northern nongovernmental organizations, foundations, and governmental aid agen-cies that provide substantial funding and services to countries where state power has been hollowed out by structural adjustment, political unrest, and corruption. Although these providers of funding and aid can enable proj-ects that might otherwise not be possible, they bring with them sets of ex-pectations and priorities determined elsewhere, in much wealthier settings, which may or may not meet local scientific priorities and protocols. The re-sult is a postcolonial science characterized by a similar "uneasy symbiosis" of collaboration and discontent.

Sherry Ortner has made the important observation that "in a relation-ship of power, the dominant often has something to offer, and often a great deal. The subordinate thus has many grounds for ambivalence about resist-ing the relationship" (Ortner 1995, 175). This is certainly the case with HIV research in Uganda, where foreign projects are welcomed as much—and usually more—than they are resisted, due to the resources and opportuni-ties they bring, as well as for the knowledge they may produce. In addition,

I would argue that this ambivalence reflects a field of power relations much more complex than the dominant/subordinate binary described by Ortner. As much as the research relations I describe in this ethnography are shaped by (and sometimes engender) steep inequalities, the story I present is by no means a simplistic tale of "subordinate" African science "dominated" by powerful Western interests (see also Tilley 2011). This is certainly not how the Ugandan researchers I spoke with viewed their situation, nor is it how the Americans envisioned their work.

Instead of a story of domination and subordination, this book tells the story of what Anna Tsing has called the "grip" or "friction" of numerous encounters (2005, 5), including those between American HIV researchers and Ugandan doctors; molecular science and clinical medicine; humanitarian aid and scientific ambition; "global" health and "local" priorities. Friction, in Tsing's formulation, is a way of describing the "awkward, unequal, un-stable, and creative qualities of interconnection across difference" (ibid., 4). Friction thought of in this way can encompass unequal power dynamics between the dominant and subordinate, but it also includes the more compli-cated relations that disrupt this simplistic binary. Yes, African biomedicine may be a vehicle for American aspirations to "do" global health, but it is also a field of knowledge and practice that actively pushes back against the for-mulation of biomedical expertise (including HIV expertise) as a Western export. As Tsing argues, "friction makes global connection powerful and effective," but at the same time, "gets in the way of the smooth operation of global power. . . . Friction refuses the lie that global power operates as a well-oiled machine" (ibid., 6).

Critical Science Studies

A central aim of this book is to interrogate the practices and politics of "global health science" through an exploration of the interplay between HIV science, technology, and global inequality. How do postcolonial poli-tics and development economics shape the production of scientific knowl-edge about HIV/AIDS? Through what mechanisms have the social rela-tions of global inequality become materially embedded within scientific technologies we use to study and treat AIDS? What are the promises and challenges of global health science in a world marked by radical inequalities between North and South? In attempting to answer these questions, I draw my principal theoretical guidance from science and technology studies and critical medical anthropology, two subfields that have both strongly influenced research and thought in contemporary anthropology, but have rarely engaged in direct dialogue with one another. My goal in fostering such a dialogue is to produce an ethnography that attends both to the social relations of science and to the political economy of health and medicine—what might be called a work of "critical science studies."

Until recently, work within science and technology studies tended to be narrow in geographic scope, with most analyses focused either explicitly or implicitly on "technoscience" in the United States and Western Europe (and, less often, Japan).[2] By mapping "science" onto the West (or global North),[3] we have been left ill-equipped to understand technoscientific knowledge production and practice in less wealthy parts of the world. I experienced this bias firsthand at a science and technology studies conference in 2005, when a senior science studies scholar responded to my research by suggesting that perhaps Ugandans were marginalized from international HIV science not because of their geographic and economic disadvantages (as I argued), but because Uganda was not a place where "good science" happened.

In recent years, cross-pollination with both postcolonial studies and anthropology has led to a welcome broadening of the geographical scope of science and technology studies. Scholars have advocated for the importance of studies of "postcolonial technoscience" and argued that "we now need to find out more about how science and technology travel, not whether they belong to one culture or another" (Pigg, in Anderson 2002, 644; McNeil 2005; Anderson and Adams 2008; Seth 2009). This shift has witnessed the

---

2. Cross-cultural studies of science did occur in the 1960s and 1970s, but tended to use "Western" science as "the benchmark criteria by which other cultures' knowledges should be evaluated" (Watson-Verran and Turnbull 1995, 115). Even critics who advocated that greater attention should be given to knowledge production in the global South tended to nonetheless implicitly locate technoscience in the North, describing knowledge production elsewhere as "other knowledge systems," "traditional" or "indigenous knowledge" or "ethnoscience"—rendering technoscience in the South largely invisible except when practiced by colonial powers (see also Nader 1996; Harding 1998).

3. Given that Africa is directly south of Europe, the global North/South distinction seems more appropriate than West/non-West for categorizing regional power differences between Africa and the United States and Europe. Nonetheless, I will at times refer to the "West," as this designation is still commonly used, and was the term often chosen by my informants.

publication of a growing number of ethnographic accounts of science and technology centered in the global South (De Laet and Mol 2000; Pigg 2001; Adams 2002; De Laet 2002; Hayden 2003; Lowe 2006; Reardon 2005; Sunder Rajan 2006; Müeller-Rockstroh 2007). These works pay serious attention to ways in which postcolonial power dynamics, including the politics of development, play out in the structuring of scientific networks and the production of knowledge. Of particular interest to my project is the light these ethnographies cast on science as a *transnational* endeavor, and the practices and processes by which global health knowledge travels in an increasingly globalized and stratified world (Petryna 2009).

The postcolonial geopolitics of illness and poverty, in which wealthy Northern countries often serve as providers of medical aid and health development funding to poor indebted countries in the South, profoundly shapes the forms that transnational biomedical science takes. For this reason, the trajectory of this book is also indebted to the large body of work within medical anthropology that seeks to understand illness and medicine as inseparable from power and inequality. The AIDS epidemic drives this point home at every opportunity, as HIV continues to travel along the economic, gender, sexual, geographic, and racial "fault lines" of society (Farmer 1999; see also Farmer and Kleinman 1989; Farmer 1992; Bourgois, Lettiere, and Quesada 1997; Pfeiffer 2002; Parker 2002; Nguyen and Peschard 2003; Fassin 2007; Biehl 2007; Hunter 2010).

Critical medical anthropology argues against the idea that disease is a freestanding biological phenomenon that exists separately from the social world. In this way, it reveals a close epistemological kinship with science and technology studies, which rejects the notion of science as autonomous from social relations. Both fields of scholarship insist upon the rigorous social contextualization of entities that are often taken for granted as objective, "natural" phenomena. Yet these fields have only recently begun to speak to one another. This is, perhaps, due to their profoundly different approaches to power and inequality. Historically, analyses of power and inequality have been mostly peripheral to science and technology studies.[4] By contrast, within critical medical anthropology, forms of social, economic,

---

4. The notable exception to this is feminist critiques of gender and science, including Martin 1991; Harding 1991; Keller 1995; Haraway 1991, 1997; and Oreskes 1997.

and political oppression, or what some have termed "structural violence" (Farmer 1997, 2003), are conceived as inseparable from illness and bodily suffering. Furthermore, public health measures or treatment campaigns aimed at redressing or preventing illness are often examined as instantiations of what Michel Foucault termed "biopower"—the control of bodies and populations through forms of management and administration (Foucault 1978). Under this analytic, even benevolent efforts to govern or improve social welfare have been theorized as forms of "symbolic violence" (Bourgois and Schonberg 2009) or "therapeutic domination" aimed at cultivating docile, self-disciplined bodies (Nguyen 2009; Rottenburg 2009).

What might a field primarily concerned with the politics of suffering and inequality and a field focused on the production of expert knowledge have to say to one another? To answer this question, we need to return to the subject of this book. AIDS, and particularly AIDS in Africa, has produced a surfeit of both human suffering and scientific knowledge over the past three decades. Moreover, these two phenomena are deeply interdependent. It is the presence of untreated illness on a massive scale that has drawn an unprecedented level of international scientific attention to Africa; and it is the desire to produce new knowledge, as well as mitigate suffering, that drives studies of HIV and other global health endeavors on the continent.

The anthropology of medicine in Africa is increasingly focusing an ethnographic eye on questions of power and knowledge production. In pursuing questions related to the ethics and politics of international biomedical research, the sociotechnical construction of bodies and maladies, and the professional, political, and moral contingencies of producing useful bioscientific knowledge and interventions in contexts of extreme scarcity and suffering, historians and anthropologists of Africa are raising crucial questions about science as a global practice in an unequal world (Gilbert 2009; Biruk 2012; Fullwiley 2011; Geissler and Molyneux 2011; Langwick 2011; Hamdy 2012; Livingston 2012). However, though a number of scholarly and journalistic works have examined the inequalities that underlie the global geography of the HIV/AIDS epidemic and its epicenter in sub-Saharan Africa (Kalipeni et al. 2003; Behrman 2004; Iliffe 2006; Fassin 2007; Epstein 2007; Thornton 2008; Mugyenyi 2008; Hunter 2010; Nguyen 2010), the production of scientific knowledge about AIDS and global health in Africa is only beginning to receive the kind of in-depth scrutiny that books such as Steve Epstein's *Impure Science* (1996) provided regarding the early years of

AIDS science in the United States. In his now-canonical account, Epstein argued that AIDS science was "impure science" because it went against the traditional notion of science as being autonomous from outside influences. This is certainly the case for global health science too, where the scientific imperative to produce data is indivisible from both the humanitarian commitment to saving lives and, increasingly, the development imperative to "build capacity" by fostering economic and educational opportunities. It is this productive but troubling nexus between disaster, assistance, and scientific opportunity that is the subject of this book.

Readers interested in the politics of global antiretroviral access and scientific debates over drug resistance in Africa and the United States will find this described in detail in chapter 1. Chapters 2 and 3 will be of interest to those curious about the molecularization of HIV medicine, the politics of technology, and the power of laboratories in global health science. The story of the research collaboration between Dr. Beale and the Wellness Center is recounted in greatest detail in chapters 3 and 4; these chapters will be of particular interest to those seeking a close ethnographic description of the power relations inherent in the practice of global health science "on the ground" and the entanglement of science, development, and humanitarianism in Africa. Lastly, chapter 5 provides a critical account of the motivations and actions of U.S. universities scrambling to create opportunities to "do" global health in Africa and elsewhere.

Opportunity and the Anthropologist: Some Thoughts on Methods

Like many of the American HIV researchers I describe in this book, my own interest in the African epidemic grew out of my experiences conducting AIDS-related research in the United States. During the late 1990s and early 2000s, I was immersed in studying the paradoxical impact of the HIV epidemic on San Francisco's urban poor, who sometimes found that an AIDS diagnosis represented their best option for obtaining stable housing and services in a rapidly gentrifying city (Crane, Quirk, and Van der Straten 2002). I was a self-identified anthropologist of urban health in North America when, as a graduate student, I was given the opportunity to spend the summer of 2003 interviewing HIV patients in Kampala, Uganda. The offer came from Dr. Beale, who was my employer at the time. Since 1999, I had worked as an interviewer and research assistant on his flagship study of HIV treatment among San Francisco's urban poor, a project that he was now hoping to replicate in Uganda. During that summer in Kampala, I got my first glimpses of the epidemic outside the United States, as well as the complicated politics of research collaboration between a very wealthy and a very poor nation. It was this trip to Uganda, along with my growing awareness of the scientific and political debates surrounding HIV treatment and drug resistance in Africa, which led me to shift the focus of my own research to the international politics and practices of AIDS science.

At the time that I began this project, I had years of experience working in HIV research in the urban U.S. but very little in the study of Uganda, Africa, or global health. My research process and the ethnographic account I have produced here reflect these disciplinary roots. This is, as many works in anthropology are today, a "multi-sited ethnography" (Marcus 1998). It tracks between multiple locations in the United States and Uganda in an effort to trace the internationalization of American HIV medicine and the growing importance of African sites, actors, and institutions in the rise of global health science. It is the in-between space of these international scientific networks, rather than the United States or Uganda specifically, that constitutes the primary "field site" of my research.

Methodologically, I approached this scientific arena in two ways: first, through participant-observation within Dr. Beale's research team; and secondly, through one-on-one interviews with North American and Ugandan HIV researchers and clinicians. My access to Dr. Beale and his collaborators and staffs in both the United States and Uganda was greatly facilitated by my status as his former research employee. Because I had worked for Dr. Beale for over four years at the time that his Uganda study became my anthropological "object," many of his U.S.-based employees working on the Uganda project were my former co-workers and friends. In addition, I made lasting friendships with some of the Ugandan research staff during the summer I spent working in Kampala. The fact that I was well known to and friendly with both the American and Ugandan research teams as well as Dr. Beale himself provided a baseline of mutual trust and respect that allowed me to gather much of the material presented here, including accounts of the group's research meetings and informal, candid conversations with study staff.

My affiliation with Dr. Beale also facilitated my access to many of the scientists and doctors formally interviewed for this research. Overall, I conducted over sixty one-on-one, tape-recorded interviews with HIV researchers and physicians for this project, roughly equally divided between Americans and Ugandans. These formal interviews were supplemented by numerous informal interviews, conversations, and observations. The formal interviews with American researchers were conducted over twelve months of fieldwork from September 2004 through August 2005, during which time I also was a regular participant-observer at meetings of Dr. Beale's U.S. research team. The Ugandan interviews were conducted during two five-week trips to Uganda in March of 2005 and June of 2009. During these trips, I was also allowed to observe meetings of Dr. Beale's Ugandan research team, as well as staff meetings at the Immune Wellness Clinic. I also conducted participant-observation at an HIV-medicine training program in Kampala that was unrelated to Beale's research. In addition, my experiences working for Dr. Beale in Kampala in the summer of 2003 provided background data for the ethnographic account I offer here.

Two aspects of my methodological trajectory necessitate further comment. First, my time in Uganda was notably brief by anthropological standards, a total of approximately four months spread out over half a decade. Secondly, I was very much a part of the international scientific network that became my primary object of study. These two factors have led me to produce an ethnography that is neither a Ugandan nor an American story per se, but rather a story of the transnational flow of knowledge, politics, research money, obligation, blood samples, viruses, drugs, and research personnel that constitute international scientific collaboration between two nations with very different histories, economies, and experiences of AIDS. My relatively short time in Uganda, as well as my immersion within the American side of the research collaboration, undoubtedly makes my knowledge of American experiences of HIV research and what I call the scientific "turn toward Africa" richer than my understanding of Ugandan perspectives. Nonetheless, I was fortunate that the "population" of scientists I chose to study was highly mobile, giving me the opportunity to conduct some of my research in Uganda, where increasing numbers of American AIDS researchers have initiated studies. While in Uganda, I gained a great deal of insight into the limits of biomedicine as a universal language—even among medical doctors—as I encountered the differences and inequalities that form the uneven terrain upon which transnational science is forged. I also worked hard to gather the reflections and experiences of Ugandan doctors and researchers treating and studying HIV. It is these perspectives that hold a sometimes grateful and sometimes critical mirror up to American research initiatives, pushing back against and resisting simplistic accounts of international science as either purely well-intentioned humanitarianism or thinly veiled neocolonial ambition.

This ethnography is structured around the experiences of Dr. Beale, and the shift of his scientific inquiry from California to Uganda. I use his experiences and those of his colleagues and employees to reflect on the opportunities and challenges raised by the rise of "global health science" more broadly. However, I could just as easily (and sometimes do) use my own experiences to make many of the arguments I advance in this book. Like Dr. Beale, I was a U.S.-based health researcher who switched my scientific (in this case, anthropological) gaze from the United States to Africa. My switch was motivated both by a desire to conduct research that might somehow contribute to improving HIV treatment access and saving lives in Africa, but also by academic ambitions that saw an intellectually exciting opportunity to study the intersection of scientific politics with social inequalities. Like many other U.S. HIV researchers, I opted to work in Uganda because that was where the opportunity presented itself and because it was a relatively peaceful country where English is a national language.[5] Moreover, like the global health research projects I describe throughout this book, my research would have been impossible without the cooperation and guidance of Ugandan colleagues. These colleagues provided not only anthropological insight, but also indispensible logistical and bureaucratic assistance to yet another American seeking to study their AIDS epidemic.

In chronicling the at times messy experiences and motivations of collaborating American and Ugandan scientists, this ethnography takes seriously the incitement for anthropology to "go beyond signaling the presence of experts and toward grappling with what kinds of persons they are" (Boyer

---

5. More accurately, the southern portion of Uganda, where most international AIDS research projects were based, was peaceful. The rural north was suffering through its second decade of a civil war against the rebel Lord's Resistance Army. The war displaced hundreds of thousands of people in the north and made traveling to that area of the country dangerous, but had little impact on the ability to conduct research in Kampala or in Uganda's southern and western regions.

2008, 39). In Dr. Beale, I was very lucky to find a scientific expert who was not only open to but actively encouraged anthropological critique of the power dynamics of international research. I can only hope that my accounts of the challenges faced by his project do justice to the complexity of these power dynamics, as well as to his deep commitment to improving HIV treatment, care, and research opportunities for Ugandan patients and health professionals. I also hope that readers will remember that any critiques I offer of his projects or other global health research endeavors are critiques that can be equally applied to my own project. My research is as much a product of the turn toward Africa and the rise of global health science as any of the biomedical research projects described in this book, and, as such, embodies many of the same aspirations and challenges.

Chapter 1

RESISTANT TO TREATMENT

As I entered the Oakwood Hotel in San Francisco's Tenderloin District, I was greeted by the incongruous scents of body odor and Indian curry. The Oakwood was one of many single-room occupancy, or "SRO," hotels populating San Francisco's Skid Row neighborhood. Originally built around the turn of the century to house unmarried and migrant industrial workers, by the late twentieth century the hotels were occupied primarily by the elderly, poor, addicted, and mentally ill (Groth 1994). Some residents established long-term homes in these hotels, redecorating their tiny rooms to their taste and paying monthly rent out of their disability checks. Others paid for only a week or two before they ran out of money, and bounced back and forth between the hotels and the street. It was the close quarters and proximity to homelessness that gave the Oakwood and other SROs their distinctive human odor. The curry scent came from the kitchens of the Indian immigrant families who owned most of the hotels and often lived in apartments on the ground floor.

I had come to the Oakwood to visit William, a young, gay, HIV-positive African American man who had lived in the hotel for the past eight years and was enrolled in the HIV research study that employed me. A native of Georgia, William still spoke with a soft Southern drawl. His small room in the Oakwood was crowded but orderly. His narrow single bed was covered in a homey afghan blanket, and the walls were decorated with birthday and Christmas cards from his family. Somewhat incongruously, a large plastic wall lamp in the shape of E.T. hung high up next to his doorway. In one corner of his tiny room, he kept a hot plate for making himself home-cooked meals. He kept a family photo album handy, and would sometimes pull it out and show me pictures of his mother and siblings in Atlanta.

My job as a research assistant was to pay monthly visits to William and other study participants taking anti-HIV drug combinations (antiretro-virals) for the treatment of their disease. During the several years that I worked for the research study in the late 1990s, I visited residents of San Francisco's SROs and homeless shelters every month to assess their "adher-ence" to HIV medications—in other words, whether or not they were taking their antiretrovirals as prescribed. Many were. William was not. As I got to know him, I came to learn that his seemingly orderly life was punctuated by periodic crack binges and, later, episodes of mental confusion. During one visit, he complained about a fractured cheekbone, an injury he told me was given to him by a "friend." Nonetheless, he was working to improve his sit-uation, and spoke excitedly about his pending Section 8 application, which, if successful, would provide him with a housing subsidy to move out of the hotel and into his own apartment.

When I asked him to show me his HIV medications, William would pull out a plastic shopping bag filled with a dozen half-filled bottles of pills. Looking at the prescription dates, I would try to puzzle out which were old and which were current. Often, the combinations of pills he told me he was taking seemed to make no sense. William himself was confused and incon-sistent about what the doctor's instructions had been, and as the jumble of pill bottles continued to accumulate in number and variety over the months, it became clear to me that he was overwhelmed. I worried that he was mix-ing pills from his old regimens in with his more recent prescriptions, and suspected that his doctor was poorly equipped to manage a patient living on the edge of homelessness, as William was. My employer, Dr. Jason Beale, an HIV physician himself, gave the doctor the benefit of the doubt and guessed that William's hodgepodge of drugs was an intentionally prescribed "salvage" regimen, a last-ditch effort at saving a patient whose virus had become resistant to multiple antiretrovirals.

William eventually moved out of the Oakwood, not because he got an apartment, but because the hotel caught fire and his room—as well as his possessions—were destroyed. After the fire, he moved from hotel to hotel. His appearance became unkempt and he became less and less mentally lucid. Finally, he returned home to his family in Georgia, where he eventually died of AIDS.

In 2003, a few years after William's death, I found myself in the back seat of a taxi in Kampala, Uganda, being interviewed by an American radio reporter. I was in Kampala for the summer at the request of Dr. Beale, who had asked me to interview patients enrolled in his new study of adherence to HIV treatment in Kampala, where antiretroviral drugs (ARVs) were just beginning to become available. For the first decade following the discovery of effective HIV therapy, the only antiretrovirals that had been available in Uganda were what one Ugandan doctor described to me as "briefcase drugs" brought back from trips to Europe in the personal luggage of the wealthy. However, by 2003 Uganda was importing ARVs from Cipla Pharmaceuticals, a generic drug manufacturer in India, and selling them to patients nearly at cost. The price was about $30 a month, and although this was still quite expensive for most Ugandans, it was much more affordable than the $1,000 a month that equivalent drugs cost in the United States (Whyte et al. 2004). Dr. Beale's study was documenting the impact of these drugs on patients' health, as well as their adherence to the regimen. The American journalist was an acquaintance of Beale's scientific mentor and a health correspondent for a nationally broadcast news program.

The reporter rode in the front seat, and awkwardly turned around and pointed her shotgun microphone towards the back where I was sitting with my colleague and friend Idah Mukyala. She had just accompanied Idah and me on a visit to a study participant named Esther, an unemployed mother of three. During our visit, Idah had surveyed Esther about her adherence to the medications, asking her questions nearly identical to those I had asked William four years earlier: "How many doses of your medication did you take yesterday? How many doses did you take the day before that?" Unlike William, Esther had only one bottle of pills, labeled "Triomune." She took only one pill twice a day. (Unencumbered by Western intellectual property rights, the Indian company had engineered a single pill containing three different antiretrovirals, a formulation not possible in the United States, where each drug was owned by a separate, competing pharmaceutical company). And also unlike William, she said she almost never missed a dose of her medication. The one exception had been just after she lost her job as a maid, when she had missed four days of the drugs because she couldn't afford to purchase a new bottle. Fortunately, she had been able to get support from a charitable organization that agreed to sponsor her medications from then on. However, she was still struggling to find enough money to buy food and to pay for her children's schooling. In words more distressing than reassuring, she told us, "It is only that I don't have a job and enough to eat—otherwise I'm not stressed anymore."[1] The visit ended with the reporter discreetly handing Esther several folded bills, uncertain of how else to respond to the situation.

During our conversation in the taxi afterwards, the reporter asked Idah and me about the research. The study that employed us was one of a growing number of projects studying antiretroviral treatment in Africa, most of which were finding very high levels of adherence to the drugs—much higher, in fact than average rates in the United States. I found myself repeating this finding into the microphone, telling the reporter that I had worked for a similar HIV treatment study back in the United States, and that people "here"—in Uganda—"take their pills more correctly than in America." Idah described how patients who owned mobile phones would set the phone's alarm twice a day as a reminder. A few months later, our words would be nationally broadcast on U.S. news radio as part of the reporter's story on HIV treatment in Africa.

That same fall, the *New York Times* published a front-page story summarizing the results of studies conducted in four countries across the African continent. The headline declared, "Africans Outdo U.S. Patients in Following AIDS Therapy" (McNeil 2003). The article described research conducted in Botswana, Uganda, Senegal, and South Africa in which patients were found to be taking over 90 percent of their antiretroviral medications. Several doctors quoted in the article emphasized that this was

---

1. See Kalofonos 2010 and Weiser et al. 2010 on food insecurity and ARV treatment in Africa.

significantly higher than typical adherence rates in the United States, which tended to be around 70 percent. These were surprising findings, as prominent health experts and policymakers had long assumed that adherence to the medications would be poor in Africa. Just two years earlier Andrew Natsios, the chief administrator of the U.S. Agency for International Development, had asserted that many patients in Africa "don't know what Western time is" and would therefore be unable to take HIV medications as scheduled (Donnelly 2001). Similar comments were made by an unnamed senior U.S. Treasury official (Kahn 2001). Because poor adherence was believed to cause the virus to become drug-resistant, a number of scientists had cautioned against expanding access to ARVs on the continent on the grounds that it could create a secondary epidemic of drug-resistant HIV. Now, by contrast, it seemed that Africans were being "made up" as "good adherers" (Gilbert 2005, 6; Hacking 1999).

The studies turned the prevailing Western assumption about HIV treatment in Africa on its head. Yet, I read the *New York Times* article and listened to my own assertion in the radio reporter's story with discomfort. It was good news that antiretroviral treatment in Uganda and other African countries was going well, but it was troubling that this finding was always presented in contrast with the comparatively poor performance of patients in the United States. Why were we so intent on framing Africans as model patients? And why, in order to do so, had I been so quick to throw American HIV patients—patients like William—under the bus?

In this chapter, I address these questions by examining the politics and science of antiretroviral therapy during the early years of the "treatment era." This was a time of great uncertainty as efforts to understand the biological mechanisms of the new drugs evolved contemporaneously with efforts to describe the risks and benefits of international ARV access. During this period, the ethical imperative to treat everyone in need appeared to be distinctly at odds with the duty to shield the public from disease threats, revealing a tension between two different forms, or "regimes," of global health (Lakoff 2010). Advocates of wider access to antiretroviral therapies invoked a global health aligned with humanitarian medicine, arguing that the scope and severity of the AIDS epidemic constituted a medical emergency and that action must be taken to alleviate suffering. In contrast, those cautioning against treatment in Africa relied upon a global health regime rooted in health security, in which drug-resistant HIV constituted an emerging infectious disease from which the world must be protected (King 2002; Lakoff and Collier 2008).

In this context, evidence suggesting that patients in Africa could (or could not) adhere or would (or would not) cultivate a drug-resistant "doomsday strain" was inherently political (McNeil 2003). Sociologist of science Dorothy Nelkin has argued that although scientific controversies typically take the form of debates over technical issues, they are often, at heart, arguments over moral and political questions (Nelkin 1995). This chapter explores two of these seemingly technical debates in an effort to foreground the political and moral questions at their cores. First, I recount the scientific and policy disputes surrounding HIV treatment access and drug resistance as they played out in relation to (first American and then African) patients perceived as unlikely to take antiretrovirals properly. Although on the surface this appeared to be a debate about medication adherence and missed pills, I argue that it was ultimately about inequality, citizenship, and Africa's relationship to globalization and modernity. Second, I explore the rise and fall of drug-resistant HIV as a potential "superbug." The perception of drug-resistant HIV as easy to transmit but very difficult to treat fed Western anxieties about antiretrovirals in Africa. However, this perception was based in part on an erroneous assumption that HIV treatment would mirror tuberculosis treatment, where poor adherence had led to the development and spread of a lethal, multidrug-resistant bacterium. As scientific understandings of the mechanisms of antiretroviral resistance developed, researchers instead found that viral resistance could develop even among highly adherent patients, and that drug-resistant virus was often treatable (though certainly not benign). Moreover, the arrival of a candidate "nightmare strain" of HIV in New York City forced a public reckoning with assumptions about the global geography of antiretroviral resistance and the framing of Africa, rather than America, as the location from which drug-resistant HIV would emerge and spread.

The chapter concludes by considering the perspectives of Ugandan doctors on the debates over antiretroviral adherence, drug resistance, and Africa. Their opinions about antiretroviral adherence and resistance among their own patients are diverse, but collectively their reflections suggest that the long-awaited arrival of internationally-funded HIV treatment in their country signaled not only new hope for patients, but a form of global recognition and inclusion for a continent still struggling for respect and legitimacy in the postcolonial era.

A Divided Epidemic

For the first fifteen years of the epidemic, HIV was a death sentence in slow motion. Initial HIV infection was typically accompanied by a bout of flu-like symptoms, followed by a symptomless period that could last for several years—even a decade—before the virus's gradual attack on the immune system led to AIDS, a syndrome marked by extreme weight loss, disabling and sometimes disfiguring infections, and other "opportunistic" illnesses, eventually ending in death. Beginning in the 1980s, doctors and researchers began testing a variety of experimental medications against the new disease, but even the most promising drugs worked only temporarily. Patients given AZT (zidovudine), the first drug to show any efficacy against the virus, initially improved, only to decline rapidly upon developing resistance to the medicine. The same thing happened with subsequent anti-HIV drugs. Researchers learned that as a retrovirus,[2] HIV was prone to rapid genetic mutation. This tendency posed a major barrier to the development of effective AIDS treatment, as HIV's mutability allowed it to quickly evolve into variants that were genetically resistant to AZT and other similar antiretroviral drugs.

This changed in the mid-1990s, when researchers developed additional classes of HIV medications that attacked the virus in new ways. When prescribed in tandem with the older drugs, these combinations—dubbed highly active antiretroviral therapy, or HAART—were able to stave off drug resistance and preserve patients' health for the long term in ways that had been previously impossible. The remarkable recovery of AIDS patients very near death following treatment with HAART was widely described as "the Lazarus effect." In the United States, the regimen's high cost—between ten and fifteen thousand dollars a year—was covered by insurance companies and the AIDS Drug Assistance Program, a federal funding mechanism

---

2. Retroviruses are viruses that carry their genetic information in the form of RNA rather than DNA.

initiated to ensure that even the uninsured could access treatment. As a result, by the end of 1996 the death rate from AIDS in the United States declined for the first time since the onset of the epidemic fifteen years earlier (CDC 1996).

Elation over the success of the new treatment dovetailed with a rising awareness of the global scope of the AIDS pandemic. Because AIDS was first documented in California and New York City, it was initially viewed primarily as an American disease, especially by those outside the United States[3] (Farmer 1992). Within a short time, however, it became clear that AIDS was global. Reports from sub-Saharan Africa, in particular, grew increasingly alarming as time passed. In East Africa, a zone of political instability and black-market trade between Uganda and Tanzania created a perfect storm for an explosive epidemic in the 1980s and early 1990s (Iliffe 2006). In the late 1990s, it became clear that southern Africa was even more severely impacted, and reports from the region began to border on the apocalyptic. In Botswana, for example, one-third of the adult population was infected by the year 2000, up from about 3 percent only a decade earlier (ibid., 39). A U.S. National Intelligence Estimate report released in January of 2000 predicted that a quarter of the population of southern Africa was likely to die of AIDS, and warned of the possibility of "demographic catastrophe" in some African nations.

Escalating reports of the epidemic's devastating effects in Africa clashed with sentiment in the United States that the discovery of HAART meant AIDS was on the brink of being conquered. In 1996 a *Newsweek* cover story ran the hopeful headline, "The End of AIDS?", and in the months that followed, HIV became increasingly described as a "manageable, chronic disease" (Leland 1996; Jacobs 1997). But not long after, reports from Africa warned that as many as one in four people might be infected in the hardest-hit countries (Altman 1998). In his ethnography of the epidemic in West Africa, anthropologist and HIV doctor Vinh-Kim Nguyen describes his personal experience of this moment in AIDS history from his vantage point in a Canadian hospital:

---

3. In some African countries, there was a running joke that the acronym AIDS stood for "American Invention to Discourage Sex" (Schoepf 2003).

I remember the first clinical trial in 1994 that used one of the new drugs—
saquinavir—in combination with two of the older drugs we used to prescribe singly. The results were stunning. In our hospital, patients stopped
dying. Some patients were literally resurrected from their deathbeds by the
new drugs. I wondered how these miraculous new treatments would get to
Africa. But in the AIDS conferences I attended, this was not discussed. The
drugs were too expensive. In Africa, it would have to be prevention and perhaps palliative care (Nguyen 2010, 3).

Indeed, the African experience of the discovery of HAART was one of
being "on the outside looking in" (Mugyenyi 2008, 96). Dr. Peter Mugyenyi,
a Ugandan HIV expert and leading advocate of treatment access in Africa,
described the sentiment at the 1996 International AIDS Conference in Vancouver as "either that of indifference or open discouragement—just in case
the Africans got carried away with ideas of introducing the highly sophisticated designer drugs to their miserable set up" (ibid). The AIDS epidemic
was dividing in two: a treated epidemic in wealthy countries, and an untreated one in poor countries. For activists and supporters of treatment, the
contrast was difficult to bear, and as the 1990s wore on advocates around
the world grew increasingly vocal about the imperative of making HIV
treatment accessible in Africa and other regions in the global South.

Initially, it was the high cost of AIDS medications that appeared to be
the primary barrier to global treatment access. With governments in the
United States and other wealthy countries struggling to cover the new drugs
at home, it was difficult to imagine funding treatment abroad. But before
too long, lower- to middle-income countries like Brazil, South Africa, and
India began manufacturing generic ARVs for domestic use and export
(Grady 2001). Sometimes described as "copycat" drugs, these pills were developed using reverse-engineering and were produced in nations where law
did not require observance of American and European patent protections.[4]
Generic antiretroviral combinations could cost as little as a dollar a day per

---

4. In the United States patent protection is granted for a period of twenty years, during which
the manufacturer enjoys market exclusivity. Only once a patent expires is it legal for other companies to make and sell generic versions of a drug. Though generic ARV production initially faced
aggressive opposition from the multinational "branded" pharmaceutical industry, it was eventually upheld by the World Trade Organization as allowable under the group's Trade-Related aspects of Intellectual Property, or TRIPS, Agreement (Westerhaus and Castro 2006).

person, and although this price was still out of reach for many individual African patients, it made the possibility of external, donor-funded treatment in Africa much more economically feasible.

In the Name of Public Health

Even as drug pricing became less prohibitive, the political will necessary to allocate aid dollars in support of antiretroviral therapy in Africa remained largely absent in the United States and other wealthy donor nations. Once global treatment became economically possible, the debate about expanding ARV access to the "developing" world, and in particular to sub-Saharan Africa, shifted to questions of feasibility at the technical and behavioral levels. In this shift, concerns about economics became reframed as concerns over global public health. First, researchers and policymakers asked, would it be technically feasible to safely and consistently administer high-cost, high-tech, multi-pill regimens in areas with limited physical and health infrastructure? And second, would patients with little education and few resources be willing and able to adhere to (i.e., "comply" with) the regimens? Concerns about consistent drug supply and adequate adherence were both rooted in the fear of drug resistance: if patients missed doses, their HIV could easily mutate into a drug-resistant strain, rendering the drugs ineffective and, as one medical journal article argued, "making the developing world a veritable 'petri dish' for new, treatment-resistant HIV strains" (Popp and Fisher 2002).

Within HIV medicine, the belief that missed medication doses would lead to viral resistance was hegemonic from early on. In the United States, anxiety surrounding antiretroviral adherence and drug resistance was fed by recent failures in tuberculosis control. In the late 1980s and early 1990s, tuberculosis rates in the United States began to climb at an alarming rate, spurred on by Reagan-era cuts to anti-TB programs and rising cases of HIV (which made infected individuals more susceptible to TB by weakening their immune systems).[5] In 1991 the TB population in New York topped

---

5. Global rates of tuberculosis and drug-resistant TB were also on the rise at this time, leading the WHO to advocate a policy of "directly observed therapy," or witnessed dosing, for TB treatment (Harper 2010).

4,000 for the first time since 1967, and many more of these cases were drug-resistant than ever before (Specter 1992). One outbreak of multidrug-resistant TB (MDR-TB) killed thirteen inmates in New York prisons (McFadden 1991).

Experts argued that resistant TB was on the rise because many patients were failing to complete the months-long regimen of antibiotics required to cure active tuberculosis, often because of mental illness, drug abuse, or homelessness. As a result, New York City began to impose enforced hospitalization on "recalcitrant" tuberculosis patients who repeatedly failed to complete their treatment. These modern-day Typhoid Marys were often patients like William: African Americans from the most marginal fringes of society (Navarro 1992).[6] Similar issues arose in other U.S. cities as they confronted their own growing rates of tuberculosis. Health officials justified the medical detention of noncompliant patients as necessary for public safety. One Denver professor of medicine put it this way: "Say I'm totally drug-resistant and I still like going to movies and I like going to restaurants and I like getting in buses and I like teaching in schools," he told a *New York Times* reporter. "If I had a gun and I waved it around in all those places you would lock me up. This is no different than a loaded gun" (Belkin 1991). This coding of incomplete adherence as a threat to not only one's own health but to the general public, as well as the public image of the nonadherent patient as poor and dark-skinned, would play a significant role in subsequent debates over the threat posed by drug-resistant HIV.

Like TB treatment, successful HIV treatment required patients to take a combination of several drugs over an extended period of time. From early on, the guidelines for HIV treatment echoed those for tuberculosis treatment and stressed the importance of assuring "near-perfect" patient adherence—95 percent or higher—as a key tool for warding off the development of drug-resistant virus (Chesney 2003; DHHS 2003). Understandably, adhering to such regimens was challenging for many patients—especially given that

---

6. Of the thirty-three tuberculosis patients detained by the NYC Public Health Dept. between January of 1988 and April of 1991, 79 percent were black, 79 percent were drug users, 49 percent were homeless, and 61 percent were men. Many were also mentally ill, and had been hospitalized for TB several times previously. Seventy-three percent had drug-resistant tuberculosis (Navarro 1992). The law under which tuberculosis patients were forcibly hospitalized dates from the era of Mary Mallon—"Typhoid Mary"—who was believed to have infected fifty people with typhoid fever prior to 1915 (Barbanel 1991).

the treatment for HIV was indefinite, with no endpoint in sight. Further-more, the "pharmaceuticalization" of HIV care that came with the develop-ment of HAART effectively sidelined broader issues such as nutrition, housing, poverty, and mental health from patient care, as the drugs came to be seen as a "magic bullet" for treating the disease (Biehl 2007). This made it easy to frame patients like William as "noncompliant" or "poorly adherent" rather than socially and economically marginalized.

Having witnessed the recent upsurge of MDR-TB, many AIDS doctors feared the development of drug-resistant strains of HIV among their poorly adherent patients, and some went so far as to withhold ARVs from home-less or drug-using patients they believed would be unable to adhere (Collins 1996; Waldholz 1996; Sontag and Richardson 1997).[7] (Indeed, Dr. Beale's initial research among homeless people living with HIV was spurred by his desire to "prove" that even the homeless could succeed on the new drugs. And, in fact, for every patient in the study who struggled like William did, there were several more who did very well on ARVs). A spirited debate en-sued as to whether this practice was a breach of the Hippocratic oath, or a professional obligation necessary to protect the public's health (Baxter 1997; Bayer and Stryker 1997; Lerner, Gulick, and Dubler 1998; Sollitto et al. 2001; Senak 1997).

Once pressure began to mount for antiretroviral treatment in Africa, similar fears resurfaced with a new international slant, shifting the locus of concern from patients like William to patients like Esther. Experts feared that antiretroviral treatment in Africa would backfire. At stake was both the health of individuals, who would gain little benefit from the drugs if they became resistant to them, and the greater public, who could be faced with the threat of untreatable, drug-resistant strains of HIV. The World Bank urged caution, asserting that "Problems with patient compliance are likely to be worse in low-income countries due to low education and the many other problems that poor people in developing countries face" (World Bank 1999, 180–181). A 2001 commentary in the medical journal *The Lancet* raised the specter of resistant virus, arguing, "Widespread, unregulated ac-cess to antiretroviral drugs in sub-Saharan Africa could lead to the rapid

---

7. Studies later showed that clinicians' estimates of who would and would not be adherent were no more accurate than random guessing (Tchetgen, Kaplan, and Friedland 2001; Paterson et al. 2000).

emergence of resistant viral strains, spelling doom for the individual . . . and leading to transmission of resistant virus" (Harries et al. 2001). This article, authored by a team of British and Malawian researchers, is typical in its focus on technology, infrastructure, and expertise—all of which were seen to be lacking in Africa. This and other scientific opinion pieces warned of the possibility of antiretroviral or therapeutic "anarchy" if HIV treatment in Africa were not carefully monitored and controlled (Horton 2000; Stevens, Kaye, and Corrah 2004). While experts who cautioned against global treatment access did not make direct comparisons between the U.S. urban poor and patients in Africa, it seems noteworthy—as Dr. Beale told me, with intentional irony—that the targets of fear remained "poor black people."

Concerns about adherence and drug resistance in Africa were echoed in the press, where writers argued that low-income African patients could not be expected to comply with the multi-pill regimens that even middle-class American patients found challenging (Sullivan 2001). "Unsupervised" distribution of antiretrovirals in Africa would be "dangerous," one physician and medical writer argued, because it could encourage the rapid emergence of drug-resistant HIV that might then "boomerang back to the West" (Mukherjee 2000).[8] This argument was picked up by the multinational "branded" pharmaceutical industry, which in the late 1990s was coming under increasing attack for its pricing practices and its aggressive efforts to block the manufacture of cheaper generic antiretrovirals in poor countries (McNeil 1998).[9] For example, the website of the Pharmaceutical Research and Manufacturers of America (PhRMA), the leading U.S. pharmaceutical industry group, made liberal use of both scientific and journalistic assertions about barriers to adherence in Africa and the associated danger of

---

8. The author of this article, Siddhartha Mukherjee, would later become a well-known medical writer, and was awarded the 2011 Pulitzer Prize in nonfiction for his book *The Emperor of All Maladies: A Biography of Cancer.*

9. In 1997 a consortium of forty branded pharmaceutical manufacturers filed a suit against the South African government—then headed by Nelson Mandela—in an effort to stop the country's production of generic antiretrovirals. Their lawsuit was supported by the Clinton administration, which, at the urging of the U.S. Pharmaceutical Research and Manufacturers of America, threatened to enact trade sanctions against South Africa (McNeil 1998). In 1999, the Clinton administration withdrew its support of the lawsuit after AIDS activists repeatedly picketed Vice President Al Gore's presidential campaign stops, chanting "Gore's Greed Kills" (Cooper, Zimmerman, and McGinley 2001). The lawsuit was eventually dropped.

drug resistance. "Unfortunately," the industry site claimed, "few developing nations until now have made public health programs a priority. In the case of HIV/AIDS, 'the therapies require taking a dozen or more pills every day at precise intervals without fail, plus high-tech monitoring for viral resistance, plus still more drugs to control side effects,' says *National Journal*. 'Try that in an African town with dirty water and mud roads'" (PhRMA 2006). In passages such as this, the barriers to AIDS treatment in Africa were strategically reframed. It was not international trade policy or corporate drug pricing that stood in the way of treating African AIDS patients, but rather Africa itself—its weak governments, lack of trained physicians, poor laboratory facilities, impoverished and malnourished patients, and "dirty water and mud roads."

Some of these worries had merit. For example, recent research conducted in Uganda has documented that some patients may miss medication doses for lack of easy access to clean drinking water in a private setting (Kawuma 2011), and new ARV distribution programs have had to devise means to ensure drug delivery in areas with few paved roads (Weidle et al. 2006; Bajunirwe 2011). Health care services in many parts of Africa are underfunded, understaffed, and undersupplied—although it is important to recognize that Western structural adjustment policies have played a considerable role in shaping this reality (Pfeiffer and Chapman 2010). Also, as I discuss in chapter 3, the laboratory technologies that are fundamental to HIV care in the United States (CD4 and viral load testing) are not available in many African health care settings. Moreover, it is well known that patients in the United States and other wealthy countries have struggled with the demanding ARV regimens and their side effects, even under the best of circumstances. However, in the U.S. context, even those who argued that denying treatment to patients like William could be justified specified that such decisions should only be made on an individual, case-by-case basis, and not on broad sociodemographic criteria (Bayer and Stryker 1997). In contrast, the argument against treating AIDS in Africa was remarkable in that it succeeded in framing the withholding of treatment from millions of people—indeed, an entire continent—as beneficial for public health. Judging by its publication in leading medical journals, this view was considered scientifically legitimate (though certainly not universal; see, for example Nkengasong, Adje-Toure, and Weidle 2004). How did this come to be?

African Time and "'Africa' Talk"

Science studies scholars have demonstrated that the sanctioning of knowledge as scientifically legitimate is deeply contingent upon the historical and social context in which truth claims emerge (Shapin and Shaffer 1987). In this vein, we can understand the successful framing of antiretroviral treatment in Africa as a threat to health security rather than a humanitarian public health imperative as dependent upon the continued social resonance of deeply held stereotypes positioning Africa and Africans outside "Western" modernity. For centuries, the dominant Euro-American imaginary of Africa has been one of a "dark continent" characterized by disorder and, in particular, disease (Vaughan 1991). Within this discourse, Africa was and continues to be seen as "the world par excellence of all that is incomplete, mutilated, and unfinished"—a foil of "absolute otherness" against which the West has constituted its own norms and subjectivity (Mbembe 2001, 1–2). The implication of African alterity (Mudimbe 1988) can be seen in expert warnings framing the continent as a place unsuitable for modern antiretroviral drugs.

This historically entrenched imaginary of African difference—"dirty water and mud roads" dysfunction, lack of "Western time,"—was handily accessible to those who argued against expanding antiretroviral treatment on the continent, and it bolstered their ability to frame the high-tech drugs as inappropriate, even dangerous, for deployment in African settings depicted as primitive. Also at work in the statements of Andrew Natsios and others was a version of what Charles Briggs and Clara Mantini-Briggs have called "medical profiling." Africans were deemed to be "unsanitary subjects," who were "incapable of adopting [a] modern medical relationship to the body, hygiene, illness, and healing" (Briggs and Mantini-Briggs 2003, 10). Placing expensive, powerful medications into such unreliable hands would be both wasteful and dangerous.

The power of this kind of discourse of difference is an instructive example of how representations of "Africa," or what James Ferguson dubs "'Africa' talk," can engender consequences independent of any relationship to empirical reality (Ferguson 2006, 2). "Africa"—always offset in quotation marks—Ferguson argues, is "a category through which a 'world' is structured" (ibid., 5). Though "Africa" conceived this way is more imagined than real, he argues, it nonetheless has very tangible and material effects: "Fantasies of a categorical 'Africa' (normally, 'Sub-Saharan' or 'black' Africa) and 'real' political-economic processes on the continent are interrelated"—for example, when negative perceptions actively discourage meaningful private investment in African economies (ibid., 7). Arguably, this was also the case with AIDS treatment at the turn of the millennium, where perceptions of "Africa" as a place of "antiretroviral anarchy" and a potential "petri dish" of drug resistance actively worked to maintain the status quo of Africa as a treatment-free zone. Moreover, what began as "'Africa' talk" facilitated the emergence of what we might call "public health talk," in which the non-treatment of a fatal illness was justified as protecting the global public's health. In this way, "Africa" is, as Ferguson says, "a category within which and according to which people must live" (ibid., 5). And perhaps, in the case of AIDS treatment, also a category according to which people must die.

It was within this discursive environment—in which the ability of Africans to tell time was publicly called into question by high-level U.S. policymakers—that the well-publicized findings that African patients were, in fact, highly adherent to antiretrovirals, emerged. The results of the adherence studies profiled in the *New York Times* and on U.S. national radio in 2003 seemed to provide righteous scientific fodder for those, myself included, who found U.S. reticence to support ARV treatment in Africa profoundly unjust. If American patients who took, on average, only three-quarters of their medications had unfettered access to ARVs, it made African patients who took nearly 95 percent of their drugs seem undeniably "deserving" of equal access to HIV treatment. In addition, science seemed to offer a redemptive narrative: the African patient—formerly seen as a danger to global public health—was now redeemed as exemplary in his or her pill-taking behavior. The former "unsanitary subject" was now a model "sanitary citizen . . . credited with understanding modern medical concepts and behaving in ways that make them less susceptible to disease" (Briggs and Mantini-Briggs 2003, xvi).

In this new scenario, it was American patients who didn't match up—a comparison made all the more damning by the fact that they were getting their drugs for free, making their missed doses seem not simple indications of absentmindedness or disorganization, but ungratefulness. "If the whole family is pooling its resources to pay for you," said one American doctor quoted in the *New York Times*, "you damn well better take your drugs.

That's a whole different scenario from the U.S., where patients get free medicine, and if they change therapy, will let a month's worth go to waste" (McNeil 2003). It was the notion of "deserving" treatment that would eventually make me uncomfortable with the *New York Times* coverage and my own brief statements about adherence on American news radio. If, as I had told the radio reporter, it was true that Ugandans took their HIV drugs "more correctly" than Americans, what did this say about American patients struggling to survive, such as William? If adherent African patients deserved treatment, did that mean that poorly adherent African American patients like William did not? Were Africans now model patients, the "worthy poor" whose diligence in taking their pills justified funding the treatment programs that kept them alive? Were impoverished American patients comparatively "unworthy" of these expensive, lifesaving drugs? Was treatment a question of merit, or of human rights? In retrospect, I see this valorization of African over American patients as a tactical move—a "politics of strategic reductionism" (Comaroff 2007). It was a gamble that treatment advocates took in the hopes that it would advance the cause of antiretroviral access in Africa without endangering treatment opportunities for socially and economically marginalized patients in the United States.

Fortunately for William, what ultimately determined his ability to get treatment was not a symbolic "sanitary citizenship" but his actual, legal membership in a country that subsidized the drugs for its citizens. As a citizen of a functioning, wealthy state, William got treatment for his HIV through a federal system designed to provide care for indigent patients— whether or not he was adherent. Although any given individual physician might have hesitated to prescribe ARVs to him, the state supported his antiretroviral treatment even as it failed to provide him with adequate care in other ways. Esther, as a member of a poor, donor-dependent state enfeebled first by colonialism, then despotism, and most recently by structural adjustment and privatization, found that her legal citizenship did her little good in treating her HIV. She, instead, was forced to turn to the "thin" citizenship that Nguyen (2005, 2010) calls therapeutic citizenship, relying on her international contacts within research projects, charitable groups, and even a chance encounter with an American radio reporter to cobble together the resources she needed to keep herself alive. At the same time, as a research subject in an adherence study framed as proof that Africans could take ARVs successfully, her exemplary pill-taking contributed to the construction

of a form of sanitary citizenship for all Africans with HIV. While this reha-
bilitation of the African patient was a boon in the fight for global treatment
access, it came at the cost of providing discriminatory health policies and
practices with scientific legitimacy. By allowing drug resistance to continue
to be framed as the outcome of individual failure, this positive re-imagining
of the African patient reinforced the same bitter logic as its negative predecessor: that some people merited treatment, and others did not.

Historicizing resistance

The public discourse surrounding ARV adherence and resistance had implications beyond the moral framing of HIV patients—it also had consequences for the symbolic framing or "signification" of the HIV virus itself
and the global AIDS epidemic as a whole (Treichler 1987). Embedded
within Western anxieties surrounding antiretroviral adherence and anar-
chic imaginaries of Africa and Africans were more subtle assumptions
about the causes, lethality, transmissibility, and geography of drug-resistant
HIV. Like drug-resistant tuberculosis, resistant HIV was understood to be
a rapid and inevitable outcome of missed medication doses. Experts described resistant virus as signifying "doom for the individual" (Harries et al.
2001, 410) and believed that it could be easily transmitted to others, thus
posing a significant risk to public health. However, drug-resistant HIV was
not always imagined as such a threat. In fact, when I interviewed HIV drug
resistance experts for this book, I was surprised to learn that there had initially been "huge skepticism" among clinicians and scientists that HIV drug
resistance would have any significant negative impact on patients at all.

When HIV was first discovered in the 1980s, the predominant view in
medicine was that viruses, once they developed drug-resistant mutations,
became too weak to replicate in the body and were thus unable to cause
disease. This belief was based on clinical experience treating the herpes
virus with the drug acyclovir. Dr. Ron Pajaro, an American HIV clinician
and nationally recognized expert on antiretroviral resistance, explained it to
me as follows:

> At that point, there was huge skepticism that anti-viral resistance was at all
> relevant to the clinic. There was one experience with herpes simplex virus. It

was common to find acyclovir-resistant virus, but acyclovir would still usually work. It was only in the rare case when it wouldn't work. And the reason for that, it was learned after a while, was that the acyclovir-resistant
viruses didn't grow very well in the body. They didn't really replicate well
enough to cause any disease. And so that was the expectation for HIV resistance.

Pajaro wanted to test this expectation, and made his mark in the field by
putting together a group of doctors and virologists to study the impact of
HIV drug resistance on patients. The team he organized analyzed the results of a large clinical trial of AZT, the principal antiretroviral drug available at the time. Their study, published in 1995, showed that drug-resistant
HIV was in fact quite different from drug-resistant herpes. AZT-resistant
HIV remained able to reproduce itself inside the body, and rendered AZT
useless in a matter of months. At the time, these findings were so contrary
to what was expected that prominent colleagues accused them of making a
mistake in their analysis of the data.

As it would turn out, Pajaro's findings would coincide with historical
events that rapidly caused the pendulum of scientific opinion about HIV
drug resistance to swing from dismissal to fear. The outbreak of MDR-
TB in New York in the 1990s and the alarm that it caused shifted the lens
through which drug-resistant HIV was viewed. Rather than comparing
HIV to drug-resistant herpes, experts likened it to multidrug-resistant TB,
which was potentially lethal and carried with it a particular image of danger marked by race and class (Bangsberg, Moss, and Deeks 2004). "HIV
drug resistance frighteningly recapitulates the history of antimicrobial drug
resistance in bacteria with a pernicious twist," wrote one prominent HIV
researcher in 2004 (Richman et al. 2004, 1398). Following the TB publicity,
Pajaro told me, the discourse "was very much the broad brushstroke that
resistant HIV is not going to respond to anything."

Once resistant HIV was framed as analogous MDR-TB, it was a short
step to figuring potentially poorly adherent patients like William and Esther as threats to public health. However, a closer examination of the history
and epidemiology of drug-resistant HIV reveals both these assumptions to
be erroneous. Tuberculosis, in retrospect, was a misleading model for predicting HIV drug resistance. Moreover, the major source of drug resistant
HIV strains did not turn out to be the urban poor in the United States or

Africa, but middle class (and often highly adherent) patients in North America and Europe.

Cracks in the conventional wisdom about drug-resistant HIV were revealed in a rather dramatic fashion in February of 2005, when the cover of the *New York Post* featured a nearly full-page headline warning of the discovery of a "nightmare strain" of HIV not in Africa, but in New York City, where a gay man in his forties was found to be resistant to all three major classes of antiretrovirals. The man had only recently tested HIV-positive and had never taken any HIV drugs previously, indicating he had been infected with a virus that was *already* drug resistant. Furthermore, his CD4 count was dangerously low, meaning he met the criteria for an AIDS diagnosis even though evidence suggested he had become infected only a few months earlier.[10] This unusual combination of multi-drug resistance and seemingly aggressive disease progression proved so alarming to the New York City Department of Health and Mental Hygiene (DOHMH) that its director, Dr. Thomas Frieden,[11] took the unusual step of holding a press conference to announce the discovery and alert clinicians and hospitals to screen their patients for evidence of the virus (City of New York 2005).[12] The New York officials' alarm was echoed in a case study of the infection published a month later in *The Lancet*, in which experts (including one of the developers of HAART) asserted that the combination of multiple drug resistance and rapid progression to AIDS made the virus "unique" and warned that "the public health ramifications of such a case are great" (Markowitz et al. 2005). At a major scientific AIDS conference that was held (coincidentally) just two weeks after news of the infection was made public, last-minute

---

10. His CD4 count was 80 cells per cubic millimeter of blood, where normal is between 500 and 1500. AIDS is diagnosed in anyone with a count of less than 200.

11. Interestingly, Frieden was involved in the investigation and combating of the MDR-TB outbreak as a CDC Epidemiologic Intelligence Service Officer and New York City's Assistant Commissioner of Health for Tuberculosis Control during 1990s. In 2009, he became the Director of the CDC.

12. The New York health officials' concern over the virus was fueled by the patient's description of his sexual activity. In the DOHMH's press release, the infected man was described as a methamphetamine addict who regularly engaged in anonymous, unprotected anal sex with other men while high on crystal meth. Calling the case a "wake-up call to men who have sex with men" and citing rising rates of sexually transmitted disease among gay men, Commissioner Frieden urged the gay community to do more to stop the spread of HIV and methamphetamine use among its members (City of New York 2005).

changes were made to the conference schedule in order to devote an entire session to discussion of the virus (Conference on Retroviruses and Opportunistic Infections 2005). The news media jumped on the story, producing multiple articles about the arrival of the potential "AIDS superbug" (Santora and Altman 2005; Perez-Pena 2005; Edozien 2005; Honigsbaum 2005).

That such a virus would arise in New York rather than in Kampala or Gabarone should not have come as a surprise. Despite expert and policy-maker anxiety over viral resistance emerging in Africa, it was well established that the bulk of HIV drug resistance occurred in Europe and North America, where treatment had been available for over a decade.[13] For example, one study of San Diego patients reported that nearly half of those on treatment had developed some degree of drug resistance during the late 1990s (Garrett 2001; Richman et al. 2004). Research also indicated that these drug-resistant viral strains were being transmitted to others. Although exact numbers are difficult to come by, a 2004 review showed that anywhere from 8 to 27 percent of newly infected (and never-treated) patients in the United States carried a virus with at least one drug-resistant mutation, and that 10 percent of people newly diagnosed with HIV in Europe showed some drug resistance (Tang and Pillay 2004). In contrast, the review included only one study of drug resistance in Africa, conducted in Côte d'Ivoire between 1997 and 2000, which found no evidence of transmitted ARV resistance.[14]

Significantly, antiretroviral resistance in the United States is most prevalent among highly adherent, well-educated, middle class, white, insured gay men, and not the homeless, mentally ill, and drug-addicted patients of color that physicians initially feared would foster viral resistance (Garrett 2001). The primary reason behind the high levels of resistance in this comparatively privileged population is not a failure to take treatment as prescribed, but rather an aggressive pursuit of effective medication in the face of near-certain death in the early years of the epidemic. Prior to the advent of HAART, it was primarily middle-class gay men and their allies who

---

13. Brazil and Argentina, both of which have long-standing antiretroviral treatment programs, also have significant levels of drug resistance.

14. Although rates of antiretroviral resistance in Africa have increased over the last decade as treatment has become increasingly available, the transmission of resistant viruses continues to be low (WHO 2011).

mobilized to demand access to experimental treatments for the disease that was devastating their communities. Having spent much of the previous decade fighting for gay and lesbian rights, this was a politically savvy and organized group—and despite ongoing homophobia, they were remarkably successful in getting their demands met (Epstein 1996; Altman 1988; Crimp and Rolston 1990). As a result, many of these patients were exposed to antiretroviral drugs one at a time as they first became available—a phenomenon doctors describe as "sequential monotherapy." This practice was unavoidable given the circumstances, but was later determined to be a perfect recipe for cultivating multiple drug resistance over time. As a result, those patients who survived into the era of HAART often harbored viruses that were already resistant to older drugs such as AZT, 3TC, and d4t. Thus, while the high level of drug resistance in this very adherent population might appear surprising from a purely behavioral perspective, it is less so when examined through a historical lens. The New York "superbug" was born from this history, as it turned out that the New York patient had contracted the virus from a Connecticut man who tested HIV-positive in 1993 and had been treated with both single and dual antiretroviral drugs prior to the advent of HAART (Blick et al. 2007).

Reimagining Resistance

The New York City case served as a reality check on the geography and epidemiology of drug-resistant HIV. But it also unleashed a scientific backlash that ultimately challenged commonly held ideas about the lethality and transmissibility of resistant virus. Even as some experts defended the decision to hold a special press conference to warn the public about the New York virus, other equally prominent AIDS scientists accused them of fear mongering, and described the case as "not a discovery", "not a surprise", "hardly unique", "not a novel finding" and "common" (Brower 2005; Cohen 2005; Smith 2005; Volberding 2005; Piller 2005; Jeffreys 2005). As time passed, it became evident that although the virus did contain multiple drug resistant mutations, it was not accurate—as the press release had reported— that it "did not respond to three classes of anti-retroviral medication." In fact, several months after the press conference the patient was doing well on therapy, though his treatment consisted of a combination of six drugs rather than a more typical three or four drug regimen. In addition, the DOHMH's claim that the patient had progressed rapidly to AIDS—perhaps "within two to three months" of becoming infected—turned out to be incorrect (Volberding 2005). Furthermore, a number of researchers expressed doubt that the virus was highly transmissible, and argued that even if it were to be transmitted to others it would likely behave differently in different patients or "hosts." They noted that similar cases of HIV had been documented in Vancouver in 2003, and that these viruses had not been passed on to others, suggesting that they were not easily spread.

This downplaying of the significance of the New York case was supported by growing evidence that drug-resistant HIV was, in fact, a little bit more like herpes and less like tuberculosis after all. For example, in the early 2000s, physicians studying the management of U.S. patients with resistance to multiple HIV drugs published data showing that many of these patients continued to do well clinically despite their mutated viruses (Deeks et al. 2000). In other words, even though testing showed them to be "resistant" to the drugs they were on, the medicines were continuing preserve their health. The reason behind these paradoxical findings, researchers argued, was that resistance mutations weakened the virus, making it less able to replicate efficiently (Barbour et al. 2002). Furthermore, these weaker viruses appeared to be more difficult to transmit to others (Leigh Brown et al. 2003; Booth and Geretti 2007), suggesting that drug-resistant HIV might also be less of a public health threat than had been initially thought. This reduced "replicative capacity" or "viral fitness" was an unexpected benefit of many drug-resistance mutations—a sort of a silver lining to an otherwise dark cloud.

The discovery that resistance mutations did, in fact, weaken the HIV virus was thus not a revolutionary finding but rather a return to earlier ideas about viral resistance. Jim Greene, one of the senior researchers who contributed to the findings about viral fitness, echoed Dr. Pajaro's comparison to herpes. "The way I think about it is: is HIV like MDR-TB, or is it like drug-resistant herpes?" he told me. "Clearly [HIV lies] somewhere in between. The latest news suggests that it's more toward the herpes side. I think more data is needed, but I think that it's more toward the herpes side." Although these findings are now widely accepted, the research was very controversial when first presented at scientific meetings. David Capelli, a young Ph.D. involved in the research on viral fitness, told me of scientific conference sessions that ended up in "shouting matches" over data:

> I think people were very concerned about what the message of our work could be. . . . We were—I think "accused" is the right word—of saying that we thought it was okay for people to have drug resistance. And that maybe it was even good news. You know, and I think even though we tried to very carefully deliver our message onto the broadest stages in the field, I think there was still active misinterpretation of that message. We were never trying to suggest that we thought drug resistance was okay.

Dr. Capelli's account of the controversy suggests that the debate over this research was moral as much as it was scientific. By implying (however unintentionally) that drug resistance might be "okay," the research upset the standard moral framing of resistance as a form of negative payback for poor adherence, and suggested that patients might instead be rewarded for missing their drugs.

Similarly provocative findings about the causes of antiretroviral resistance were also emerging at this time, as research results began to challenge the conventional wisdom that poor antiretroviral adherence inevitably led to the rapid development of drug resistance (Bangsberg and Deeks 2002). In a study of antiretroviral treatment among U.S. HIV patients, researchers found that drug resistance was most concentrated among *highly* adherent patients—those who took nearly all of their doses as prescribed—rather than those who frequently missed their pills (Bangsberg et al. 2003). In other words, in some cases, "near perfect" adherence seemed to encourage rather than prevent antiretroviral resistance. Also surprising was the finding that patients with the worst adherence (under 65 percent) had little drug resistance, though they also had little clinical benefit from treatment. The researchers explained their paradoxical findings by arguing that the relationship between poor adherence and drug resistance had been overly simplified in the scientific literature and was, in fact, different for different types (or classes) of HIV drugs. For certain older classes of antiretrovirals, missed doses did in fact lead rapidly to drug resistance, just as most researchers and clinicians had long believed. But for the newer protease inhibitor[15] class of drugs, over half of all resistance appeared in patients with the best adherence to their medications (those who were 79 to 100 percent adherent in the study), and particularly among patients who took most—but not quite all—of their medicine. Though initially counterintuitive, the researchers explained these results as a factor of different drug-specific "genetic barriers" to resistance.[16] Given the common belief that it was poor adherence that caused drug resistance and "near perfect" adherence that prevented it, these findings were provocative. In addition to upsetting the conventional wisdom in HIV medicine, they also complicated the moral calculus established during the MDR-TB outbreak that linked poor adherence, "recalcitrant" patients, and dangerous, drug-resistant disease. Paradoxically—on some regimens—it was the model HIV patients who were developing drug resistance.

Although this research was conducted in the United States, these and other related findings about differences across classes of HIV drugs were very relevant to then-nascent efforts to expand antiretroviral access in Uganda and other African countries. The older antiretrovirals were chemically simpler drugs than the newer protease inhibitors, and this made it easier for generic drug companies in India and elsewhere to reverse engineer and manufacture them. They were also much cheaper. As a result,

---

15. It is important to note that ARV therapy has improved since the time of this study. Protease-inhibitor regimens are now routinely supplemented or "boosted" with a low dose of ritonavir, an ARV that improves the efficacy of the anchor protease inhibitor and reduces the risk of resistance. Most of the participants in this study were not on "boosted" regimens.

16. Mutation only occurs when the virus is replicating. Ideally, perfect adherence keeps drug levels in the blood high enough to prevent the virus from reproducing, thus also stopping it from mutating. However, when drug levels drop—perhaps due to missed doses—the virus may begin to replicate again. When HIV replicates in the presence of an antiretroviral drug (under what scientists call "drug pressure") the mutations that develop are likely to be resistance mutations, as it is these genetic changes that give the virus the ability to "escape" the drug. HIV can become resistant to some older ARVs by undergoing a single mutation, but it must mutate many times in order to become resistant to a protease inhibitor. In the study, patients who took less than 65 percent of their protease inhibitors had levels of medication in their blood that were simply too low to push the virus to accumulate the numerous mutations needed to develop resistance. For these patients, it was essentially as if they were taking no medication at all. But in patients who were highly—but not quite perfectly—adherent to protease inhibitor-based regimens, drug levels dipped low enough to allow viral replication but stayed high enough to force the virus to mutate in order to do so, creating the perfect pharmacokinetic conditions for the development of drug resistance.

when HAART started to become more widely available in Uganda—first through the importation and sale of generics (primarily Cipla's Triomune), and later through international aid programs—regimens were almost exclusively comprised of combinations of the older medications. While equally effective, these combinations were much less "forgiving" of missed doses (Crane 2007; Thompson et al. 2010).

The pitfalls of this reliance on older combinations were not lost on African doctors and experts. In 2005 I sat in on an HIV-medicine training course held in Kampala. The course was intended to help prepare doctors from Uganda and other nearby countries for the increasing numbers of patients on antiretroviral drugs under their care.[17] During one presentation on drug resistance, a visiting Canadian lecturer described how different antiretrovirals had different thresholds for resistance, and pointed out that HIV could become resistant to the drugs nevirapine and lamivudine (commonly called 3TC) following a single viral mutation. "So," he told the class, "you'll realize immediately—what's the most common drug in Africa?" *Triomune*, the class answered—the Indian-manufactured combination pill containing both lamivudine and nevirapine, as well as a third drug. "So, two drugs with very little genetic barrier. Why?" he asked the class. *Because it's cheap*, they accurately responded. At this point the doctor seated behind me noted to herself, "Uh-oh. We're in trouble." One Ugandan expert I spoke with later described HIV treatment in his country as "a question of money"—in other words, what people and programs could afford to buy. The older drugs in Triomune had been rendered affordable by generic manufacturers, whereas protease inhibitors (which remained largely under the control of branded pharmaceutical companies) had not. As a result, despite earlier Western anxieties about drug resistance in Africa, the antiretrovirals that eventually made it to the continent first were often those most likely to cause resistance the quickest if doses were missed.[18]

Although epidemiologic data on the emergence and development of HIV drug resistance in Africa remains limited, the extremely low availability of

---

17. The course was organized by the Infectious Disease Institute at Makerere University, which I describe in chapter 3.

18. This disadvantage is somewhat offset by the comparative simplicity of the older combinations, which generally contain fewer pills than protease-inhibitor regimens, and are thus sometimes easier to adhere to. Both kinds of regimens are considered HAART.

antiretrovirals in Africa prior to 2005 means that drug resistance on the continent is low (Sendagire et al. 2009). The resistance that does exist can often be linked to "triage"—drug pricing decisions, health policies, and acts of desperation, like medication sharing—that have resulted in incomplete and interrupted treatment. For example, during the decade following the discovery of HAART, treatment in most of Africa was limited to those with sufficient money to buy medication, connections to procure drugs from abroad, or who were lucky enough to gain enrollment in a research study (Whyte et al. 2004; Nguyen 2010; Epstein 2003).[19] But these sources of drugs were often unreliable or unsustainable. In 2005, Dr. Gregory Odong, a physician from northern Uganda, described the problem to me:

> People started getting the drugs many years ago. But not from Uganda. People in Uganda initially had the benefit of going out [of the country]. Some went out on asylum. Now as they made contacts outside, they also got into contacts with people who could provide the drugs. So there we have briefcase drugs, which were being siphoned into Uganda.

Dr. Odong told me that these people either took the drugs themselves or gave them to relatives in need, but usually with little to no medical supervision or advice. As a result, they did not know which drug combinations to take. These were "the most difficult lot of people" for HIV physicians such as himself, as they were the ones who showed up at major referral hospitals like his, suffering from drug resistance. "They already tried almost every kind of drug combination," he continued, "and some have run out of options now." Later, as generic and discounted drugs became available, additional pathways to viral resistance arose in Africa, as patients bought ARVs when they could afford to do so but, like Esther, missed doses when they could not (Weidle et al. 2003; Adje-Toure et al. 2003; Byakika-Tusiime et al. 2005).

Because Andrew Natsios's words about African adherence and drug resistance had been such a lightning rod for the debate over global treatment

---

19. Botswana is an exception to this. Through a partnership between the government of Botswana, the Gates Foundation, and Merck Pharmaceuticals, ARVs were available through Botswana's public health system somewhat earlier, beginning in 2002 (Carpenter 2008; Brada 2011a).

access,[20] I asked Ugandan doctors I interviewed for their thoughts about his assertions. Their reactions were more varied than I anticipated, and revealed ambivalence about both African adherence and African modernity. Although several doctors described his comments about Africans and "Western time" as "paternalistic" or "offensive," one young medical officer at the Immune Wellness Clinic in Mbarara told me that she thought fears about antiretroviral resistance emerging in Africa were "warranted" because "most of the Africans, especially the ones who are not educated, they're not so time-conscious." One of her colleagues at the clinic similarly argued that while studies in Uganda had "disproved" Western fears concerning adherence in Africa, "You could say they had a good reason to think about it, because [of] issues like illiteracy, poverty, and everything. When you have someone and they don't have a watch, he can't know what time to take his medicine."

In Kampala, Dr. Tabitha Byakika, a prominent expert in pediatric AIDS, told me that worries about poor adherence were "obviously a consideration for us even as African researchers and clinicians." Like her American colleagues, she cited earlier experiences with failed tuberculosis treatment as a cautionary tale. However, she did not view the risks as a reason to withhold treatment. "The issue of resistance has always been there, even in the West," she told me. "[But] the benefit of antiretrovirals is so significant . . . we couldn't say we're going to worry about a theoretical risk when people are actually dying from HIV." Dr. Byakika thus saw Western fears about adherence and resistance in Africa as a valid scientific inference based on the challenges of TB treatment, but a flawed basis for policy. Other Ugandan experts, however, disputed the scientific legitimacy of such fears on the basis that very few studies of antiretroviral adherence in Africa had actually been done at the time. For example, Dr. Joseph Muhwezi, a senior researcher in Kampala, told me that "as a scientist working here, you really get angry many, many times when people express sentiments of that nature that have no scientific or any other evidence base."

---

20. Even the American radio reporter who accompanied Idah Mukyala and me on our research visit in 2003 made a point of asking Esther, the patient, how she knew when it was time for her to take her HIV medications. Her response—"I just look at my clock"—was featured in the broadcast story as an explicit rebuttal to Natsios's claims.

Some Ugandan doctors dismissed the statements by Natsios and other experts as "ignorant." In interviews, they repeatedly expressed the sentiment that such ideas were misconceptions that could only be expressed by someone who had not spent time in Africa (although, in fact, Natsios had traveled there extensively). For example, one young physician and aspiring researcher in Kampala described the comments about time-telling as a "stereotype" stemming from "people who have never probably been to Africa. "These were researchers sitting on boards, making decisions, making these kind of comments," he told me. Dr. Mary Balenzi, an Mbarara physician who would later become director of Mbarara's Immune Wellness Clinic, told me "I found [the debates] quite insulting." Nonetheless, she said, "I don't blame them very much because some of them wouldn't know what is happening in Africa, when you're there and you've not been here at all."

"It was a lack of knowledge" that allowed such statements to be made, she argued, and "a perception of Africa which is like we're down, down on the globe. Like really we are down to the dogs."

Dr. Ezra Mukasa, an elderly but spry expert on pediatric AIDS, was the most outspoken regarding the ignorance of Americans. It was "clear," he insisted, "that most people who talked about Africa, and Africans not adhering to this, had never been to Africa. This is a terrible thing! You cannot judge somebody without knowing him. Their view of Africans are the American Negros, who are extremely different from Africa. Extremely different!" Here Mukasa appeared to be challenging American stereotypes of Africa by invoking his own seemingly negative assumptions about black Americans. He went on to comment on the low social position of black men in America, noting that he rarely saw them at the numerous scientific conferences he had attended in the United States. "You hardly find any African American [men] there," he told me. "These days we find a lot of women, so women are making up. And men, I don't know where they are." In this expert's words we see the same logic employed by the media reports that touted the superiority of African adherence over that of American patients. Mukasa simply made the racial component of this discourse explicit.

A senior professor of medicine in Kampala, Dr. Mukasa originally hailed from the rural Rakai District in southwestern Uganda. Rakai is home to a long-standing HIV research project affiliated with Makerere and Johns Hopkins universities, and the research done there has been the subject of numerous conference presentations and scientific publications. Mukasa worked and traveled in the international scientific circles where this research was presented. Raising his voice, Mukasa described his anger upon encountering what he saw as an unfair representation of his home district at an international medical conference:

> I remember, in one conference somebody showed a residence of one of the persons in the Rakai district. And I was there. And I protested. [Imitating the voice of the presenter] "Oh, this is their homestead of these people living in Rakai." I told him, "Yes, you've been to Rakai, but I was born there. Is this the real house people live in? How many houses have you visited?" He started blushing because he did not know that among the audience there were people who come from there. . . . It was too poor! It was a shack. Somebody who did not even have a door. I would not say that people even ever lived in that place at all.

It was not that Dr. Mukasa thought his country was wealthy. Earlier in our conversation, he recalled bringing American visitors to the home he had built outside of Kampala, a place he described as "a very beautiful building overlooking the city." When the visitors complemented his house, he responded by reminding them that it was "an exception."

"There are very poor people in this country who live in shacks. And there are very rich people with big houses, even bigger than where I'm living now," he said. "So you can only say that different people live differently."

Thus, the issue of African poverty was a complex one for the Ugandan doctors I spoke with, who struggled to counter Western perceptions of Africa as "down to the dogs" with the reality that they were elites living in an otherwise poor country. Even Dr. Mukasa's statements were somewhat contradictory, first denying that someone in Rakai would actually live in the "shack" depicted at the conference, but then later remarking that there were "very poor" people in Uganda who did, in fact, live in "shacks." In Mbarara, a young medical officer complained to me, "People of the West just have this general idea that Africa is still a very dark continent, that we are like monkeys basically." But her objection to this bigoted view was hardly a statement of African pride: "I think we are somewhere," she insisted. "I know we are backward, but we are somewhere."

In this way, the Ugandan experts and doctors I spoke with struggled to negotiate what Ferguson has described as Africa's "perverse" relationship to globalization, characterized by "highly selected and spatially encapsulated forms of global connection combined with widespread disconnection and exclusion" (Ferguson 2006, 14). On one hand, it is the so-called modernization of Africa in the form of urbanization, industrialization (especially mining in the south), and increased human mobility that is believed to have initially allowed AIDS to shift from a local, endemic disease in central Africa in the mid-twentieth century to the continental epidemic (and global pandemic) it would become by the turn of the millennium (Iliffe 2006). The social and demographic shifts that would eventually carry HIV along paved roads, trading corridors, migrant labor routes, battle lines, and airline flight paths developed alongside African independence and efforts to forge modern, self-governing nations out of territories of disparate polities that had been arbitrarily grouped together via colonial conquest. In addition, these changes contributed to the development of an urban, cosmopolitan elite in many African countries. In Uganda, it was this elite—and particularly its doctors—who would bear the chief political responsibility for confronting the country's AIDS epidemic (Iliffe 2002, 220). But in doing so, this elite wrestled with the formidable challenges they faced in fighting AIDS in their impoverished country, and sometimes invoked pessimistic and primitivist imaginaries of Africa not unlike those deployed by Western skeptics of treatment access.

Perhaps not surprisingly, for Ugandan HIV doctors and researchers the high adherence rates documented among their patients was a source of pride. It bolstered not only their hopes for the success of antiretroviral therapy in Uganda, but also Africa's claims for inclusion in the world of global HIV medicine. The discovery that antiretroviral adherence in Uganda and other African countries actually surpassed rates in the United States challenged age-old stereotypes of Africa as a "dark continent" of "dirty water and mud roads," a place that was "down to the dogs," where people "lived like monkeys" and didn't understand "Western time." It was poor, but it was *somewhere*, and it had promise, if only given a chance. The ability to take what were seen as some of the most high-tech, cutting-edge pharmaceuticals in the world—and take them properly—thus signaled a kind of membership in the global community, and a challenge to Africa's exclusion from it.

This membership was further signaled by the long-awaited arrival of free antiretroviral therapy on the continent. United Nations Secretary General Kofi Annan's call for an AIDS "war chest" led to the founding of the Global Fund to Fight AIDS, Tuberculosis, and Malaria, which began disbursing international donations to fund antiretroviral treatment in poor countries in 2002. Even more surprising was U.S. President George W. Bush's 2003 announcement of his President's Emergency Plan for AIDS Relief, or PEPFAR, during his January State of the Union address. The plan allocated $15 billion dollars over five years to support antiretroviral therapy in some of the world's hardest-hit countries, primarily in Africa.[21] Together, these initiatives would usher in the start of Africa's "treatment era." As I describe in chapter 3, the programs would have a profound impact on HIV treatment and research in Uganda.

As antiretroviral drugs become increasingly available in Africa, drug resistance on the continent will rise (Gupta et al. 2010). This fact has much more to do with medication access than it does with medication adherence (Crane et al. 2006). The relative scarcity of antiretroviral resistance in Africa reflects the historical lack of treatment in African countries, just as the high rates of drug resistance in the United States stem from the longstanding availability of ARVs in wealthy nations. In this way, global inequalities in treatment access have become manifest as biological differences between individuals who have received full treatment, partial or inadequate treatment, and no treatment at all (Nguyen 2010, 105). Such a reading resists the framing of viral resistance as primarily a factor of individual pill-taking behavior, and instead suggests that the epidemiology of drug resistance—like the epidemiology of HIV itself—represents an embodiment of the history of treatment access and, more specifically, "the embodiment of inequality" (Fassin 2003). Like other forms of drug resistance, its emergence is rooted as much or more in politics and markets than in individual pill-taking behavior (Orzech and Nichter 2008). Understanding HIV drug resistance as

---

21. The politics behind the founding of PEPFAR have been the subject of much speculation, and lie beyond the purview of this book (see Behrman 2004 for one account). Possible motivations for the program's announcement include post-9/11 worries over the destabilizing effect of AIDS on African nations viewed as potential harbors for terrorism; President Bush's evangelical Christian beliefs (perhaps evident in his description of PEPFAR as "a work of mercy" in his State of the Union address); and an effort to soften the blow of his intention to initiate the war in Iraq, which was also announced in the same speech.

the embodiment of unequal treatment access requires that we reject the low prevalence of antiretroviral resistance in Africa as simply "good news." Certainly drug resistance is undesirable, and its prevention is a worthy endeavor. But the low level of drug resistance in Africa cannot be separated from the fact that the continent's epidemic went largely untreated for the first full decade of the HAART era. This lack of treatment may have prevented the development of resistant virus, but it also enabled millions of deaths from untreated AIDS. Researchers have estimated that HIV treatment saved over 3 million years of human life in the United States between 1989 and 2003 (Walensky et al. 2006). This finding suggests that many millions more years of life were lost during this period in Africa, where infection rates were much higher and treatment access much lower. Indeed, one study estimated that the lack of access to antiretrovirals in South Africa alone was responsible for the loss of 3.8 million person-years of life in that country between 2000 and 2005 (Chigwedere et al. 2008).[22] The rarity of HIV drug resistance in Africa is a reflection of this dark history.

---

22. This was not only due to pharmaceutical pricing, but also due to former South African President Thabo Mbeki's controversial embracing of "dissident" or "denialist" AIDS science, and his skepticism over whether HIV was the cause of AIDS (Fassin 2007; Mahajan 2006).

Chapter 2

The Molecular Politics of HIV

Viruses are peculiar organisms. Their structure consists of little more than a small package of genetic material (DNA or RNA) surrounded by a protein exterior called an envelope. Unlike plants or animals, viruses do not eat, drink, photosynthesize, or excrete. Unable to reproduce on their own, they are dependent upon the metabolic processes of the organisms they infect in order to replicate. Biologists have debated whether they actually meet the criteria to be categorized as living beings, describing them as organisms that "verge on life" (Villareal 2004, 103). At the same time, viruses are ubiquitous and—quite literally—a part of us. One thing that scientists discovered upon completing the Human Genome Project in 2003 was that the human genetic map is littered with the fragments of viruses. This is because certain types of viruses, including HIV, bear the distinct ability to copy and paste their own genetic material into the DNA of their host cells and have been doing so throughout human evolution. These fragments, now inert, persist inside the cells in our bodies as what was dismissed until recently as "junk DNA."[1] As a result researchers estimate that, all told, human beings are about eight percent virus (Specter 2007).

The expansion of scientific knowledge about viruses and their relation to humans is inseparable from advances in genomics and molecular biology. Knowledge about HIV, perhaps the most-studied virus in history, is no exception. In 1984 scientists published the first partial genetic map of the yet-to-be-named virus, focusing on the portions of its nine genes that would best allow comparison with similar viruses (Hahn et al. 1984). In 2009, researchers produced the first map of HIV's genetic sequence in its entirety (Watts et al. 2009). During the twenty-five-year interim between these two scientific landmarks, HIV medicine was transformed from a primarily clinical and palliative practice into a heavily molecularized field of science. Currently, in the United States, many tests and medications used in routine HIV care are engineered based on very detailed, codon-by-codon[2] knowledge of the virus's genetic material.

The use of the term "mapping" to describe this kind of genetic knowledge and practice is more than metaphorical, as the knowledge that is generated by genetic sequencing is essentially spatial, telling scientists the order and location of the molecules that make up the viral genome. In addition, mapping genes and mapping territory serve many of the same purposes: both provide a means of orienting one's self, a way of generating coherence, and a way to establish relationships between things (Rheinberger and Gaudilliere 2004). Critical geographers have long argued against "representationalism," in which maps are accepted as objective and straightforward depictions of space. Rather, maps should be understood as socially and historically contingent, and, as David Turnbull argues, as expressions of power (Turnbull 2004). In this chapter, I aim to show that this argument holds for genetic maps as well.

For example, in his study of the colonial mapping of India, geographer Matthew Edney describes how mapmaking allowed the British to transform a disparate collection of empires and territories into the single, coherent

---

1. In 2012, a large federally funded project called "Encode" (for Encyclopedia of DNA Elements) published research showing that most "junk" or non-coding DNA actually plays a critical role in regulating and controlling genes (Kolata 2012).

2. A codon is a group of three adjacent bases in a strand of DNA or RNA. Codons provide genetic code information for particular amino acids.

entity of "British India" (Edney 1997). These maps then became rapidly
naturalized, rendering the exclusions involved in constructing British India
invisible. The representation of the territory as it appeared on colonial maps
thus became taken for granted, unquestioned—the map and the territory
became synonymous. Matthew Sparke has described how alternative, "con-
trapuntal" cartographies may, in turn, upset the coherence of such naturalized maps (Sparke 1998). And Turnbull has made a direct link between
cartographic and scientific knowledge, arguing that maps are "an apt meta-
phor for scientific discourse. Scientific representations of the phenomenal
world are, like maps, laden with conventions, which are kept as transparent,
as inconspicuous as possible" (Turnbull 1989, 9).

If we interrogate how a map is constructed, we are able to understand
the partiality and contingency of its representation. We are able to understand how the map is *productive* of certain possibilities—certain forms of
understanding—and better able see what was necessarily included and excluded in order to produce a standardized entity. In Edney's analysis, this
coherent entity was British India. In my analysis, I aim to show what was
excluded in order to create a coherent, standard map of the HIV virus and,
by extension, drug resistance. My point is that the generation of coherence
(a standardized map of the HIV virus) has resulted in a situation in which
the genetic sequence of a particular strain of HIV—"subtype B," a variant
found mainly in the United States and Europe—now serves as the common
template for understanding and studying HIV worldwide.

In this chapter, I describe how these particular viruses from the United
States and Europe came to be so central to HIV science, and argue that the
implications of this fact are at once clinical, epistemological, and political.
Though current antiretroviral regimens thankfully appear to work well
against all viral subtypes, some scientists view their universal efficacy as
"lucky" and fear that future drugs, diagnostic technologies, and vaccines
designed using subtype B virus might work less well on other strains. Clinically, this presents the possibility of an antiretroviral pharmacopoeia that
could be prejudicial not only in pricing, but also in efficacy. In addition, the
ability to measure and treat drug resistance in viruses other than subtype B
may be compromised by the comparative scarcity of molecular knowledge
about how resistance emerges and evolves in the global South.

Epistemologically and politically, the story I tell here illustrates an important but perhaps little-explored link between science and technology

studies and the political economy of health. By tracking the evolution of HIV science, I argue that the geopolitics of the AIDS epidemic is present at the molecular level, in the laboratories where our knowledge about the molecular biology of HIV and antiretrovirals is produced. The result is a kind of "molecular politics" (Rose 2001) in which the global inequalities of the AIDS epidemic are manifest at the most minute scale, embedded within the very materials and tools scientists use to study HIV. This chapter is an examination of those molecular politics and their relationship to the politics of antiretroviral treatment access described in chapter 1.

Producing Coherence

Virological and molecular biology research on HIV and its treatment have traditionally focused on the genetic "strain" or subtype of HIV found predominantly in North America, Europe, and Australia. As a result, this virus, known as "subtype B," has been used to establish nearly all of what is known about antiretroviral treatment and drug resistance (Jülg and Goebel 2005; Brenner 2007). In fact, there are more than ten different genetic subtypes, or clades, of HIV, and those responsible for the lion's share of the African epidemic (as well as the global epidemic as a whole) have received little scientific attention until very recently. Instead, scientists have generally relied upon a handful of viruses isolated in American and French laboratories during the first years of the epidemic as the "reference strains" upon which their work is based. The geographic and genetic specificity of these strains is important because the development of antiretroviral drugs, the definition and measurement of drug resistance, and key diagnostic technologies used in patient care are all contingent upon genetic mapping and molecular modeling of the HIV virus. In other words, medical knowledge gained from familiarity with these viruses may not always accurately reflect the "non-B" HIV strains that constitute nearly 90 percent of the world's infections (Spira et al. 2003).

Understanding how and why this came to be necessitates a brief foray into HIV biology. The HIV virus is highly error-prone in its replication process, meaning that it mutates rapidly and constantly as it reproduces. Each viral offspring differs slightly from its parent by several mutations. This means that any given individual infected with HIV is carrying a *population*

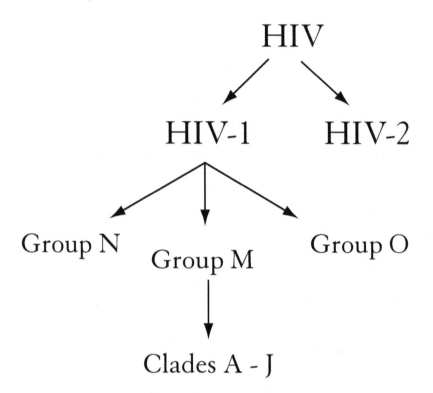

Figure 2: HIV genetic variation.

of genetically different but closely related viruses, rather than genetically identical copies of a single virus. For this reason the scientific literature refers to HIV as a "quasispecies," meaning a mixture of genetic variants of a virus, as opposed to a single virus with a consistent genome. This extreme diversity means that generating coherence is one of the key challenges involved in working with HIV in the laboratory. The result is that the need for a genetically consistent, workable virus often takes precedence over approximating HIV as it exists "in nature."

However, despite its diversity, some HIV viruses are more similar than others. The relatedness, or phylogeny, of HIV viruses is based on genetics. Viruses are mapped and grouped according to the similarity of their genetic material, which is understood to reflect their evolutionary proximity. The basic phylogeny of HIV is depicted in figure 2, which shows both HIV-1 (the most common virus) and HIV-2 (found in West Africa), as well as various groups and

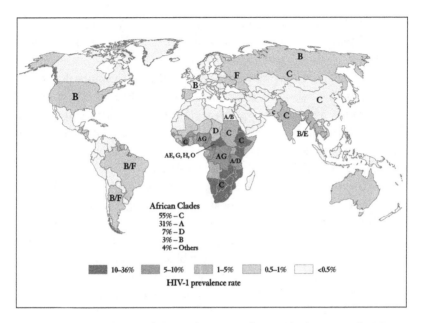

Figure 3: Subtype diversity of HIV-1 infections prevalent worldwide (Spira et al. 2003). Reproduced courtesy of Oxford University Press.

subtypes of HIV-1. In common parlance, general references to "HIV" are more accurately describing HIV-1 Group M, which accounts for 99 percent of the world's infections. There are currently at least ten identified genetic subtypes of HIV-1 group M. The first nine subtypes are each identified by a different letter of the alphabet. The tenth subtype includes several "recombinant" viruses that are actually mixtures of more than one subtype, such as A/E. (Sometimes these circulating recombinant forms are each counted as a separate subtype, making the total number of subtypes somewhat variable.)

The prevalence of these subtypes also varies geographically. In the United States, Western Europe, Australia, and parts of Latin America, the vast majority of infections are subtype B infections. Because it has the oldest HIV epidemic, sub-Saharan Africa encompasses a much greater diversity of different subtypes, with the most common being C and A (Iliffe 2006; Kantor and Katzenstein 2004). Worldwide, the most prevalent subtype is type C, which accounts for 47 percent of infections globally. This is because type C predominates in the areas of the world that bear the greatest burden of infection—particularly southern and eastern Africa (see figure 3).

Thus HIV is not one virus, but many. The ability to understand HIV at the molecular level—to literally make the genomics of the virus legible—is what has allowed scientists to understand the breadth of the virus's diversity. However, this exquisite familiarity with the details of HIV genomics also creates certain tensions in relation to generating knowledge about the virus. Specifically, scientists confront the fact that there is no single viral sequence that represents HIV. There is no unity to HIV, no standard code. This presents problems for scientists who must choose a virus to use when conducting basic research, developing drugs and vaccines, and designing diagnostic technologies. Furthermore, this viral diversity presents a problem of comparison—a particularly important element in the assessment of drug resistance. A patient's virus is tested for resistance by comparison to a virus known to be drug-sensitive. This drug-sensitive virus then serves as a standardized "reference strain" against which the patient's virus can be assessed. But given the incredible diversity of HIV, and thus the virtually infinite number of drug-sensitive viruses in existence, how is a single virus chosen to serve as a common referent?

The Contingency of the Arbitrary

Martha Lampland and Susan Leigh Star have argued that the establishment of a standard is both highly contingent and profoundly local, and the standardization of HIV certainly evidences these characteristics (Lampland and Star 2009). David Capelli, one of the American scientists I interviewed regarding HIV drug resistance and viral fitness, described the choice of reference strains to me as "somewhat arbitrary."

"In fact," he continued, "the idea that there was a normal strain of HIV is sort of strange to begin with. There really is not. It exists as a population. It's sort of like saying, 'What is the representative American?' Well, I don't know. It's a highly diverse country." In choosing a reference strain to work with, scientists selected from viruses already available to them in their laboratories; in the United States and Europe these viruses were all of the subtype B variety, as this was the strain infecting the vast majority of local patients. Many HIV researchers are physicians who first encountered the virus in their medical practice. As such, the choice to focus their research on subtype B virus reflected both its convenient availability and the desire to work on the strain that was infecting the patients under their care. However, it is important to recognize this convenient and arbitrary choice as both historically specific and socially contingent. The uptake of subtype B viruses as the basis for HIV laboratory research and technology development was not random, but reflects the fact that the great majority of both research funding and infrastructure are located squarely in the United States and Western Europe, where subtype B predominates. The result was the establishment of a reference strain that represents only 12 percent of worldwide infections (Kantor and Katzenstein 2004).

Interestingly, convenience shaped not only the choice of subtype B virus as the reference strain, but also a very specific virus within this subtype. The most commonly used reference strains are closely related and go by a number of technical names, including NL4-3, HXB2, and LAI. This proliferation of names is a product of the complex and contentious history of the virus's discovery. Capelli explained it to me as follows:

> So its full name is pNL4-3. And you mention that to basically any lab scientist who works with HIV-1 and they go, "Oh, L4-3." It probably is the basic reference virus used in North America. It's a well-characterized strain and people understand it. . . . The history on this—this would be, I think, a good thing to look into. Basically, these are some of the earliest isolates that were grown in the 1980s. And they were some of the earliest variants. So as you know, in the very early stages of the epidemic there was (A) some confusion over what was the causative agent and then, (B) once it was determined that it was HIV-1, there was a great deal of energy put into determining how to appropriately grow and sustain these viruses. And some viruses grow better in culture than others. And NL4-3 was one that did. They also called it HXB2 or LAI . . . And my understanding is that these viruses are all highly related and came from a handful of labs in the 1980s.

The labs that Capelli refers to are those of Luc Montagnier and Robert Gallo. In the early 1980s, these two scientists were at the forefront of the search for a virus that could be the cause of AIDS: Montagnier at the Institut Pasteur in Paris, and Gallo at the National Cancer Institute in Bethesda, Maryland.[3] Both scientists were specialists in the study of retroviruses—a

---

3. It was not at all obvious that AIDS had a viral cause, and during the early years of the epidemic a wide variety of other causes were considered (see Epstein 1996).

family of viruses that carry their genetic material in the form of RNA rather than DNA—and both thought that a retrovirus could be the cause of AIDS, a hypothesis that turned out to be correct. In the early 1980s, both labs worked to isolate a retrovirus from patients who were suffering from AIDS. The relationship between the labs was competitive, but they nonetheless exchanged samples according to common scientific etiquette.

In 1983, Montagnier's lab isolated a previously undocumented virus from a patient with lymphadenopathy, the swollen lymph nodes that are one of the hallmarks of AIDS. He named the virus "lymphadenopathy-associated virus," or LAV. Soon thereafter, the lab isolated similar viruses from patients with more advanced disease. One of these viruses—from a patient identified only by his initials "LAI"—was particularly fast-growing and aggressive. However, the Montagnier group's attempt to describe the virus in greater detail was stymied by the difficulty of culturing it in the lab. The virus was troublesome to grow because it killed all the cells in which it was cultured within a matter of days, and once the cells were dead, the viruses died, too. After much trial and error, the French scientists developed a technique of transferring the viral cultures to fresh cells every three days over the course of several weeks, a laborious process that would eventually yield them enough virus for further laboratory studies (Garrett 1994).

Shortly after Montagnier's discovery, Gallo's lab also isolated a virus from a patient with AIDS. They named the virus HTLV-III, believing it to be related to a group of human t-cell lymphotropic viruses, or HTLVs, that Gallo had discovered in the late 1970s (it was later determined to be unrelated). The American and French groups agreed to compare their viruses and, if they were found to be the same, to hold a joint press conference in which they would co-announce the discovery of the virus that caused AIDS (Gallo 2002; Rainey 2006).

What happened next initiated a controversy that would drag on for nearly a decade. Before the viruses could be compared, Margaret Heckler, the U.S. Secretary of Health and Human Services, held a press conference to announce that the AIDS virus had been discovered. At the conference, Gallo was heralded as the discoverer of the AIDS virus, a title he embraced. Montagnier's team was not invited to the press conference, nor was their work cited. Gallo did not dispute that Montagnier had isolated a virus earlier than he had isolated HTLV-III. Rather, he defended himself as the discoverer of the AIDS virus by arguing that it was on the basis of his

HTLV-III research that the definitive causal link between the virus and the syndrome was established, and that a blood test could be developed. Gallo's claim was boosted by his team's development of an "immortalized" cell line that did not die when cultured with the virus, eliminating the tedious culturing process used at the Institut Pasteur and providing a technology key to the development of the AIDS antibody test (Garrett 1994). On the same day the press conference was held, Gallo filed a U.S. patent application for a blood test that would identify infection with the virus. The U.S. government granted him the patent—worth $100 million annually in sales and $100,000 to Gallo personally—and denied a patent to the French (Rainey 2006).

The Institut Pasteur challenged the patent, beginning a protracted struggle between the French and the Americans that would eventually involve both heads of state. Gallo continued to assert that HTLV-III was the virus that caused AIDS, and opposed the 1986 renaming of the virus "HIV" (human immunodeficiency virus) by the International Committee on the Taxonomy of Viruses (Epstein 1996). However, a genetic analysis of both viruses later revealed that they were essentially identical. This confirmed long-held suspicions on the French side that the isolate that Gallo had "discovered" was actually derived from Montagnier's aggressive LAV/LAI virus, which is now believed to have contaminated Gallo's samples as well as those in a number of other labs with which Montagnier had shared cultures (Montagnier 2002; Gallo 2002). Eventually, U.S. President Ronald Reagan and French Prime Minister Jacques Chirac declared the two scientists co-discoverers and agreed to split the patent proceeds. Today, Montagnier is generally recognized as the first to identify the virus, while often Gallo is credited with solidifying the link between the virus and AIDS and developing the technology that made the AIDS antibody test possible (Rainey 2006; Stine 2004). Nonetheless, it was Montagnier and his colleague Françoise Barré-Sinoussi who were awarded the 2008 Nobel Prize in Medicine for the discovery, with Gallo conspicuously excluded.

Ultimately, it was the LAI isolate of the virus and its derivative copies or "clones" that would go on to become one of the most commonly used viruses in HIV research. Interestingly, LAI was not selected on the basis of its representativeness. In fact, most scientists I interviewed readily agreed that the reference strain they used was not very similar to the type B viruses most often found in patients (much less to the other non-B subtypes). Rather, these strains were used because they grew well under laboratory conditions. Having undergone genetic changes over the course of numerous manipulations in Paris and Bethesda, these viruses were now what scientists call "lab-adapted." Paula Leigh, the associate director of a nonprofit California virology laboratory, explained it to me as follows:

> Whatever the first virus that Gallo or Montagnier isolated, that's a lab-adapted strain. And it was grown out in the laboratory in vitro and propagated. And maybe even cloned out. And those are viruses that generally replicate very, very easily. You can grow them easily, that's how they found them in the first place. And they might actually be quite different from what is actually growing in people.

She then went on to give her understanding of the complex nomenclature behind the reference strains:

> LAV is the original virus that they isolated. And they call it different things depending where in the world you are—LAV, LAI, BRU, HTLV-III. And then there's another reference strain called NL4-3 which is actually a hybrid virus from two patients [that somebody] isolated and they spliced together and it's just used as a reference virus because it grows very well in tissue culture. . . . [And] there's another one, HXB2. It's often used as a reference strain and . . . is just like LAI, I think, but there's a slight difference from it.

Ralph Ernst, a Swiss scientist working at a university-affiliated blood bank in California, echoed Leigh's assessment that the reference strains were "different from what is actually growing in people." He told me, "Not only did people use subtype B, they probably used the wrong subtype B. People basically used what they had. And the first thing they had was the cloned viruses—the one that Gallo/Montagnier isolated, HXB2. So everybody kind of uses a very limited set of the oldest virus. Why?" He then answered his own question, "Because they're convenient. Everybody's got it. You can compare data across labs."

It was this ease of use, rather than the virus's representativeness, that made the LAI virus "the right tool for the job" for these scientists (Clarke and Fujimura 1992; see also M'charek 2005 for a similar case in population genetics). Representativeness, in this context, was less important than availability and suitability to laboratory conditions. A virus that was genetically more similar to the viruses in patients could have been chosen, but might have been difficult to grow in the lab.[4] In addition, once the LAI strain and its cousins had become the common currency of lab work, switching to a different reference strain was impractical because it would impede the comparison of data between laboratories. Jim Greene, a University of California virologist, put it most succinctly when he told me: "This is an example where consistency is more important than being right." After all, he continued, "there is no way to be right." In his view, it was more important for scientists to be explicit about which reference strain they were using and to be consistent in this choice than to use a reference strain that more closely resembled those occurring in patients. Greene's words reflect an important but perhaps counterintuitive characteristic of standards: the fact that they are "always already incomplete and inadequate" (Lampland and Star 2009, 14).

To be sure, this is not a new issue in science. In fact, this twenty-first-century story carries many echoes of laboratory work performed a century earlier, when *Drosophila melanogaster*, the common fruit fly, established itself as the first standardized laboratory creature during the early years of experimental genetics at Columbia University in New York. Much like the HXB2 and NL4-3 viruses, *D. melanogaster* became an integral part of laboratory practice not through calculated consideration but because it was easily accessible to urban U.S. biologists and because it was "hardy," meaning able to survive and flourish in the laboratory environment (Kohler 1993). Over time *D. melanogaster*—like the HIV reference strains—became so commonly used that it established itself as the "standard fly" for use in genetic research, even though by then it had evolved to be quite different from flies found in the wild. As Robert Kohler has argued in his account of the *D. melanogaster* story, once established, a standard organism becomes very difficult to replace or alter due to "what evolutionary biologists call a founder effect: the more elaborate the machinery of experimental production that was built around it, the more costly it would be to replace it with other

---

4. See Landecker (2000) and Skloot (2010) for an interesting comparison to the case of the HeLa human cell line, which was also rapidly taken up by scientists because it was easy to cultivate in the laboratory but, unlike HIV reference strains, became both personified and racialized through connection to a human "donor," Henrietta Lacks.

species" (Kohler 1993, 309). This was most certainly the case with HIV reference strains as well.

Molecular Economies

In its role as reference strain, subtype B virus (and specifically the LAI-related strain) has come to serve as a proxy for the otherwise highly diverse HIV genome. As such, it provides a standardized "map" of the virus in which a variable genetic code is momentarily stabilized, with particular genetic sequences affixed to a specific location on the HIV genome. This stabilization can be seen in the notation used to describe drug-resistant mutations in the virus, where a normal or expected genetic sequence is juxtaposed with a mutant or variant code. This is an extremely useful scientific tool for navigating a microbe notorious for its powers of rapid mutation, and one that has allowed scientists to develop a common language for discussing and describing HIV genetics. Consequently, subtype B became the template upon which nearly all the laboratory and much of the clinical knowledge about HIV has been based. This includes everything from the molecular models scientists have developed to understand the virus's structure to the antiretroviral drugs that have transformed the lives of patients able to access them. It also includes knowledge about drug resistance, which is defined according to mutations found in subtype B viruses.

I first learned about the significance of subtype in a 2004 discussion with Eileen Jacobs, an industry scientist who was working on developing a new test for HIV drug resistance for her employer, a multinational molecular diagnostics company. The company was already a major manufacturer of viral load assays, tests that measure the level of virus present in a patient's blood and are a routine diagnostic used in clinical practice in the United States. It was looking to expand into the market for HIV genotype assays, which can show whether a patient's virus has mutated to become drug-resistant. Our interview was one of the first I conducted during my fieldwork, and my understanding of the science behind HIV genotype testing was still very limited at the time. Assuming that the technical challenge in genotyping had to do with the large number of antiretrovirals in use, I asked her if it was difficult to develop a test that could detect resistance to numerous different drugs.

Her answer surprised me. The challenge lay not in tailoring the test to the drugs, she told me, but in tailoring it to the virus. A key element of the genotype assay, Jacobs explained, is the use of polymerase chain reaction (PCR) technology to "amplify"—make many copies of—the virus's genes. PCR works through the use of what are called "primers": these are genetic sequences that attach to the beginning and end of a targeted region of a gene, bracketing off the portion to be copied. These primers, Jacobs told me, were all initially designed based on a subtype B reference strain. As a result, they were sometimes less effective in attaching to and amplifying the genetic material of viruses of other subtypes. In the past, this had caused problems for the company's viral load test, which also uses PCR technology and was initially not very good at measuring the presence of non-B virus in patients' blood. The company had successfully reworked the primers used in the viral load assay to make it work with multiple subtypes (clades) and was now trying to do the same for a genotype test. Jacobs explained:

> Clade B is most common in this country. And so originally we knew most about that clade because that's where we could get our sequence information, that's where we could do the testing. So that's where the primers have been designed towards. So it's easy to amplify clade B. It's more difficult to amplify every clade. . . . So all the commercial tests have been developed for clade B.

In order to develop a genotype test that could accurately assess viruses from different subtypes, Jacobs's company needed to provide its scientists with non-B viruses to work with. Because the corporation was not involved in any significant international research collaborations, these samples had to be purchased from a biological supply company based in Miami. Paradoxically, the fact that these viruses were so peripheral to HIV laboratory science in the United States had ended up rendering them a commodity.

The AIDS researchers I spoke with described the field's reliance on subtype B reference strains as problematic but essentially benign in motivation—a "historical fluke" and an issue of convenience, not favoritism. Nonetheless, these and other HIV scientists were also very much aware of the limitations posed by relying so heavily on one strain of the virus, and emphasized the importance of conducting more research on non-B viruses. In addition, some also acknowledged that at a higher level, market forces were at play (see also Cooper 2007). James Briswell, a university-based expert in HIV drug resistance and non-B viruses, described the situation in terms reflecting the political economy of the global pharmaceutical market:

> Well, I think there are two reasons [why subtype B has been used]. I think one is just that it was the most convenient. People had all those subtype B samples available. And all the studies were done with B because it's in the United States and Europe. So that's more of a benign explanation. But there's no question that a lot of drug development is targeted to parts of the world where you know people are more likely to be able to pay for drugs. There could have been a lot of work done with tuberculosis and malaria, and many new drugs developed during the same time period. But they weren't because it just wasn't considered a high enough priority on the part of some of the pharmaceutical companies from people who are looking at their bottom line.
>
> So I think it's a combination. It's just that all the strains that people had in the labs were subtype B, and I think a lot of researchers just tend to work with the same strains. They're not always aware of the variability. But I think there's also an element of companies targeting the strains that infect the people in the parts of the world that have the most money.

Whether or not the *initial* choice of these subtype B viruses for laboratory research was a matter of convenience, they are now chosen by necessity. These lab-adapted strains have become established as the common referent or template for HIV research, and to change the template (by, for example, choosing a subtype C reference strain) would make it impossible to communicate with other laboratories or to compare data. It would make science "too chaotic" in the words Briswell, who told me that even researchers in the developing world—where subtype B is rare—speak in terms of subtype B:

> You almost need a common frame of reference to describe things. Even if it's arbitrary . . . just to facilitate communication. So it has nothing to do with favoring one subtype over another. It's really just a matter of convenience that a lot of the people in the field—you have to pick something as a reference. And in the future you know maybe things will change. But people are used to speaking in terms of subtype B. *No matter where you go in the world, even if they have all subtype C, they're used to speaking in terms of subtype B,*

from the literature, you know. . . . I don't think that's detrimental in any way. Because if you had people using different reference strains it would just be too chaotic. [emphasis added]

Thus, subtype B has become not only the molecular template upon which all HIV medications and diagnostic technologies are based, but also the lingua franca of AIDS research globally—even though other strains are much more prevalent. As a standardized scientific form, these viruses have achieved "irreversibility" (Callon, in Lampland and Star 2009, 14). In this way subtype B operates almost like a colonial language, allowing communication across different groups and across geography, but also reflecting a very specific and unequal arrangement of power. The power embedded in a standardized "language" is by no means limited to this instance, and can also be seen in examples as diverse as musical notation (Revuluri 2007) or the "ASCII imperialism" inherent within computer character set standards (Pargman and Palme 2009). However, the case of HIV science is notable in the potential implications it carries for health around the globe.

Consequences, Clinical and Political

Clinical researchers and clinically applied anthropologists will rightly be concerned with the relevance of the story told above to patients seeking and undergoing HIV care, and may wonder about the extent to which this reliance on subtype B impacts antiretroviral treatment and drug resistance in patients infected with "non-B" viruses (that is, most patients in the world). This is not a question that can be answered definitively, as HIV scientists have only recently begun turning their attention toward subtype differences, and the field is rapidly evolving. Nonetheless, there are some important findings thus far (see Taylor et al. 2008 for a summary). For example, research has shown that some subtypes may be more aggressive than others, leading more rapidly to death when untreated. One 2006 study of subtypes A and D, the two most common clades in Uganda, found that those infected with subtype D died an average of two years earlier than those with subtype A virus (Laeyendecker et al. 2006). This finding was reported in Uganda's leading daily newspaper under the blunt headline, "HIV Type Determines How Fast You Die" (*New Vision* 2006). Other research has suggested that some subtypes may be more easily transmissible by particular routes than others.

Historically, the research arena in which HIV subtype has drawn the most attention is in vaccine development.[5] When they announced the "discovery" of the AIDS virus in 1984, virologist Robert Gallo and HSS chief Margaret Heckler made the optimistic prediction that a vaccine would be available within two to five years. This prediction proved to be dramatically inaccurate, and twenty-five years into the epidemic the prospect of an effective vaccine is pessimistic. HIV clades have been a source of controversy in vaccine science because it is likely that preventative vaccines designed using one subtype may not work (or will work less well) against other subtypes.[6] This is because these vaccines are made using proteins from the exterior "envelope" that encases the HIV virus, which is the portion of viral anatomy with the greatest genetic variation across clades. The earliest attempts at vaccines were indeed subtype-B specific, leading to politically and ethically volatile situations when they were brought to non-B developing countries for clinical trials (Craddock 2007). Ralph Ernst, the blood bank virologist, warned me about this after I posed several questions to him regarding subtype:

> You've got to be careful [about] the political aspect of the whole trend of your research. Because there was a big concern from Africans that "Oh, you guys in the developed world, you're going to make a vaccine against subtype B and it's not going to work for us. So you're not thinking about us." You know, they have a point. Now people will make a vaccine against subtype B because that's where the money is, sadly enough.

Uganda was one site where early vaccine research caused such a controversy. The country hosted the first HIV vaccine trial in Africa in 1999, a Phase I

---

5. More recently, developers of vaccines against the human papilloma virus (HPV) similarly had to grapple with the global diversity of HPV subtypes (Muñoz et al. 2004).

6. The relationship between HIV subtype and vaccine development is complex and varies depending upon the type of vaccine under consideration. Subtype is most relevant to the development of preventative vaccines, which, like traditional vaccines against polio or smallpox, aim to stimulate an antibody response that prevents an individual from becoming infected upon exposure to the virus. Subtype is less relevant to the development of therapeutic HIV vaccines, which do not prevent infection but rather aim to inhibit viral replication and thus slow disease progression (AIDS Vaccine Advocacy Coalition 2005).

study of a subtype B vaccine. Because Uganda's epidemic is primarily comprised of subtypes A and D, this caused some concern that Ugandans were being used as "guinea pigs" for a vaccine that might not benefit them (a concern possibly augmented by earlier controversies over ethically questionable U.S.-funded AZT research in the region; see Mugerwa et al. 2002 and Wendland 2008).[7] However, this controversy was ultimately overshadowed by another: widespread fears (based on misinformation) that exposure to the vaccine would cause study participants to become infected with HIV (Kaleebu 2005).[8] In part as a result of these early controversies, there was a move to place greater emphasis on the development of non-B vaccines and "multi-clade" vaccines designed to work against multiple subtypes. This shifted the balance of research such that vaccines based solely on subtype B are now a minority of those in development (Kahn 2003).

In addition, African countries have become increasingly involved in vaccine trials. In 2000, a group of African AIDS experts convened in Kenya and adopted "The Nairobi Declaration: An African Appeal for an AIDS Vaccine." This document pledged support for increased African involvement in vaccine development and urged industrialized countries and international donor organizations to increase their financial and technical contributions toward vaccine research for Africa, "paying particular attention to the variability of HIV strains between different regions of the world" (AfriCASO 2000). Under the auspices of the World Health Organization, the group established the African AIDS Vaccine Programme to further promote and support the development of African vaccine research.

A few of the Ugandan scientists I interviewed for this research were involved in vaccine studies, some for subtype B vaccines and some for multiclade vaccines. Ronald Ntege, a leading Ugandan researcher responsible for

---

7. It is important to note that in many instances, this kind of cross-clade vaccine testing is actually a good thing. In fact, testing candidate vaccines against "unmatched" strains is crucial to determining the extent to which subtype impacts vaccine efficacy, an important issue in the development of a broadly effective vaccine (Kahn 2005). What is problematic is the fact that clade B vaccines dominated these early efforts, when B virus accounts for only 12 percent of worldwide infections. A more justifiable trial, for example, might have tested a clade C vaccine against Uganda's A and D subtypes (as is currently underway), but at the time, clade B vaccines were the only vaccines under development.

8. These early vaccines did not cause research subjects to become infected with HIV, but they did sometimes cause individuals to test positive for HIV antibodies.

some of the first studies of the epidemic in his country, was circumspect about the issue of subtype when I spoke with him in 2005. "The knowledge we have now is that really a vaccine is likely to be successful if it is tailored to the circulating subtype in the population as much as possible," he told me. At the same time, he said, it was understandable that Western companies working on vaccine development would work on the subtype that prevailed in their countries. "One has to go to look at the other side," he told me, "and say, look, most of these companies which have invested billions and billions are operating in countries where there's only basically one subtype. So they are in a dilemma." Interestingly, for Ntege even a subtype B vaccine study could be beneficial for Uganda, as it provided an opportunity to build research infrastructure and train local scientists:

> I mean we did a study which was based on subtype B and I know we heard a lot of arguments like that—"Why is it a subtype which is not [here]?" But we told them, "Look, there's something we can benefit. We can build infrastructure. We can train people. And as technology moves, we'll get vaccines based on our subtypes."

Here Ntege points out an interesting and important connection between research and development in Uganda. I refer here not to the "R&D" of the pharmaceutical industry, but rather "development" that operates in the name of advancing the social and economic lot of poor nations, or, as James Ferguson writes, the "dominant problematic or interpretive grid through which the impoverished regions of the world are known to us" (Ferguson 1994, xiii). What Ntege implies is that a vaccine study is not simply a vaccine study, but also a means by which to improve laboratory infrastructure, train researchers, and establish links with Western colleagues and funding bodies, a phenomenon I examine in detail in chapters 3 and 4. In light of these tangible forms of development—or "capacity-building," as it is often called in international health—the issue of subtype matching may be less important. Indeed, given the lack of clinical success in HIV vaccine research thus far, the capacity-building aspects of vaccine research may actually be the primary benefit that vaccine studies have to offer at the current time.

In contrast to vaccine research, subtype differences have only recently become a topic of concern within the science of HIV treatment and drug resistance. The growth of interest in the study of subtype differences is likely a result of the fact that large numbers of patients infected with non-B viral subtypes are now being exposed to antiretrovirals for the first time through the Global Fund and PEPFAR-funded programs that began rolling out free HIV medications in low-income countries in the mid-2000s. In addition, as the epidemic has become increasingly globalized, the number of non-B infections in North America and Europe has risen (Thomson and Najera 2001). Because the most effective antiretrovirals are the product of "structure-based" drug design, in which drugs are tailored to their target at the molecular level, these shifts have sparked concern within the scientific community over whether antiretrovirals designed to target subtype B might be less effective against other viral subtypes (Spira et al. 2003, 235; Atlas et al. 2005; Kinomoto et al. 2005; Holguin et al. 2006; Fleury et al. 2006). Fortunately the answer so far seems to be no, with the caveat that relevant data remains limited (Braitstein et al. 2006; Kantor 2006; Taylor et al. 2008). As treatment is scaled up in low-income countries, people with non-B virus seem to be responding to and benefiting from existing antiretroviral drugs just as well as people in the United States and Western Europe, a result that James Briswell described to me as "lucky." This is good news for patients, but raises the question: should the universal efficacy of HIV drugs be a question of luck? Of course, luck has long been recognized to play an important role in scientific discovery, and in this way the story of HIV drug development is nothing out of the ordinary. Yet the question of whether the use of more diverse research materials might lead to different kinds of "lucky" findings seems relevant.

Furthermore, as the molecular targets of HIV drugs become more diverse, the question of whether *new* drugs will work equally well across subtype is an important one. The first decade of effective HIV treatment relied on drugs that targeted two specific areas of the viral genome, interfering with the virus's ability to replicate itself. In the second decade of HAART, new drugs have emerged that target different areas of the virus, such as an injectable medication called enfuvirtide, which helps block the entry of HIV into human cells, and raltegravir, a drug that interferes with the virus's ability to integrate its genetic material into the DNA of host cells. These drugs represent two entirely new classes of antiretrovirals. If the areas of the viral genome targeted by these drugs vary highly between subtypes, it is possible that newer classes of drugs might work better against some subtypes than others.

This question arose at a 2004 conference presentation given by Françoise Brun-Vézinet, a prominent French AIDS scientist. Brun-Vézinet delivered a well-attended talk on drug resistance in non-B viruses at the 2004 Interscience Conference on Antimicrobial Agents and Chemotherapies, a major infectious disease conference held annually in the United States. During the question-and-answer period, a member of the audience of physicians and scientists asked her whether anything was known about the efficacy of the newer classes of drugs in treating non-B infections. She told the audience that although there had been initial skepticism that enfuvirtide worked against non-B viruses, a recent study had proved that it was indeed effective (see Holguín et al. 2006). But, she added, for the other new drugs [referring to drug classes under development at the time], "I'm afraid that subtype will affect it very much." In general, much remains unknown about the performance of newer drugs against non-B viruses, as they were designed and approved based on clinical trials in American and European patients who had spent years on HIV treatment and developed resistance to numerous drugs—a category that currently describes very few individuals in the lower-income countries where non-B viruses predominate. Furthermore, the small amount that is known is based on *in vitro* studies conducted on non-B viruses in the laboratory, which may or may not represent the clinical reality of how these drugs behave in patients (Taylor et al. 2008).

Lastly, I return to the question of HIV drug resistance. Drug resistance is directly related to drug efficacy, in that antiretrovirals will be less effective against viruses that have mutations causing drug resistance. To date, despite expert fears that Africa would become a "petri dish" for drug-resistant HIV, the vast majority of research on antiretroviral drug resistance has been conducted on patient populations infected with subtype B virus. This reflects not only the (now shifting) geographical bias of AIDS research, which initially focused much more on the epidemic in North America and Western Europe, but also a technological bias in that the tools used to test for drug resistance were designed to do so in subtype B.

Researchers and clinicians use two different methods to assess whether a virus has become resistant to antiretrovirals: genotyping and phenotyping. Genotype testing is the cheaper and most commonly used option (and is the technology that Eileen Jacobs' company was working to improve such that it could adequately amplify non-B viruses). Genotyping works by comparing the genetic code of a patient's virus to that of a drug-susceptible reference strain, which serves as a genetic map of what the virus "should" look like if it has not mutated to become drug-resistant. However, because the canonical reference strains are all subtype B viruses, scientists are uncertain about whether they serve as an accurate yardstick by which to gauge drug resistance in other viral subtypes. For example, a genetic configuration that is defined as a resistance "mutation" in a subtype B virus might actually be normal or "natural" in another subtype (Jülg and Goebel 2005). In addition, because resistance mutations have been defined based on genetic changes observed in subtype B viruses, much less is known about what resistance might look like in viruses with different (i.e., non-B) baseline genetics (Martínez-Cajas et al. 2008). As of this writing, there is no evidence that the *interpretation* of any given resistance mutation differs across subtype: in other words, a mutation that commonly causes drug resistance in subtype B virus will have the same result in a subtype C virus. Where differences do exist are in the patterns of mutation across subtype, meaning that some genetic changes are more common in some subtypes than in others, and that different viral subtypes may take different genetic pathways to drug resistance. The clinical implications of these differences for patients, if any, are still unknown (Geretti 2006).

Concerns about subtype have also arisen in relation to the phenotype assay, which is a costlier but more direct test for drug resistance than genotyping. Rather than looking for genetic mutations, phenotyping involves exposing a patient's virus to different drugs in the laboratory in order to see which drugs are able to stop the virus from replicating. Importantly, phenotype tests do not use a patient's virus in "whole" form, but rather graft the relevant genes from a patient's virus into a standardized viral vector, which is then exposed to a series of antiretrovirals *in vitro*. Because these standardized vectors are derived from the classic subtype B reference strains, HXB2 and NL4-3, some researchers have expressed concern that they might limit the accuracy of phenotype testing in assessing resistance in non-B viruses (Geretti 2006; Martínez-Cajas et al. 2008; Wainberg and Brenner 2012).

There is currently no smoking gun showing serious differences in drug resistance across subtype. However, further studies of non-B subtypes are considered an important priority within the field and differences are "increasingly emerging" as research evolves (Kantor 2006). For example, in clinical studies of the prevention of mother-to-child transmission of HIV, subtype C seems to develop resistance to the drug nevirapine more rapidly than other viral subtypes. This is worrisome because nevirapine has been widely used in Africa both to impede perinatal HIV transmission and as a key drug in combination therapy regimens. At the same time, laboratory studies of new integrase-inhibitor drugs suggest that subtype C viruses may develop resistance to these medication *less* easily than subtype B viruses—a finding that, while interesting, seems unlikely to have much impact on HIV care in Africa due to the high cost of these new formulations (Wainberg and Brenner 2012).

It is only recently that these questions of difference have become a topic of significant scientific inquiry. The reasons for this, as I hope I have made clear, rest in the interrelationship between the molecular politics of HIV research and the political economy of antiretroviral treatment access. Early on in the epidemic, viruses reflecting the genetics of HIV in the United States and Europe were integrated into laboratory research and rapidly became the lingua franca of molecular virology. For many years, these reference strains remained an unmarked category—a universal template for HIV genetics. The choice of these strains was both born out of and served to perpetuate the near-exclusive focus of HIV treatment and drug-resistance research on clade B virus. Furthermore, the lack of access to ARVs outside wealthy subtype B countries made research beyond these parameters difficult and unlikely, as it meant that there were very few patients with non-B virus undergoing antiretroviral treatment, and thus very few in which the effects of treatment—including drug resistance—could be effectively studied.

The push to roll out ARVs in Africa and other low-income regions of the world changed this picture. Confronted with a global epidemic comprised mainly of subtype C and other non-B viruses, scientists began to confront the fact that their laboratory reference strains were not unmarked or universal but were, in contrast, very specific viruses with particular histories and genetic cartographies. They were, in short, artifacts with embedded politics (Winner 1980). The result has been a growing awareness of and interest in differences in treatment and drug resistance across geographies and subtypes. However, due to the newness of these inquiries, a great deal remains unknown. Comparative studies often tend to lump all non-B viruses together, making it difficult to determine how, for example, the subtype C viruses that predominate in South Africa might act differently than the subtype D viruses prevalent in Uganda (Holguín et al. 2006).

And research possibilities continue to be constrained by the optimization of resistance tests to subtype B reference strains and the paucity of non-B viral sequences in the HIV genetic databases used to identify resistance mutations (Wainberg and Brenner 2012). "The data," Ralph Ernst reminded me in 2005, is still "so slim. People don't do serious drug-resistance studies in non-B countries, or they've done very few of them."

It seems important to juxtapose the "slimness" of this data with the broadly stated conjectures about HIV drug resistance in Africa described in the previous chapter. Those conjectures were made in the absence of any significant data on drug resistance in Africa, yet they played prominently in policy debates over whether or not treatment should be expanded in Africa. And, significantly, such debates continued to haunt the field even after the political tides turned in favor of treatment access, as James Briswell told me in 2005:

> I think a lot of people who are involved in this drug-resistance research in Africa and Asia, like I am, are concerned that [the research] will be taken out of context, and people would exaggerate this fear [of resistance] and use it as a reason not to give therapy. That's a major concern among experts in drug resistance that fears of resistance not be blown out of proportion, so that they're not looked at as a reason not to give therapy.

Scientists are in agreement that the data on non-B drug resistance is scant and needs to be pursued in greater depth. There are an increasing number of researchers committed to this agenda. Yet, as Briswell describes, they conduct their inquiries with the fear that the data they are beginning to collect may be interpreted as a reason not to further expand treatment in poor countries—an expansion they greatly support. This fear seems to indicate that despite the major shift in international will toward support of antiretroviral treatment in Africa, fear of drug resistance has retained a powerful political valence.

In addition, it is important to note that the research into non-B drug resistance is still centered in wealthy industrialized countries, where the technology exists to conduct the molecular analyses involved in drug-resistance research. Uganda, despite its prominence in other areas of AIDS research, such as epidemiology and prevention, is "rather thin" in the field of biological research, as one Ugandan epidemiologist put it to me. Training more

Ugandan molecular biologists, he thought, would lead to more drug-resistance research on Ugandan HIV clades:

> Molecular biology is rather thin. I was talking to somebody who was trying to pursue a career in the laboratory sciences and I said, "Just go for molecular biology." [In] the epidemiological sciences, I think we have trained a sufficient number of epidemiologists. Behavioral scientists are being trained. Laboratory scientists are being trained. But molecular biologists and virologists, immunologists, those are in short demand. So, the only way we could develop, [that] we could study drug resistance working on our clades, is by developing the capacity ourselves. I think that will be easier.

Like Ronald Ntege, this scientist made a link between research and capacity-building. If Uganda had greater local research capacity—particularly within fields like molecular biology, he argued—more research on clades relevant to Uganda would be done. This seems a fair prediction, given that biologists often base their work on clinical samples available from local patients. It also raises the important question of how molecular knowledge about the virus might have evolved very differently had the global centers of scientific power laid elsewhere.

How We Know

This chapter began with a discussion of cartography, in which I argued that maps are socially constructed representations of a territory based on the specific inclusion and exclusion of different types of information. Over time these representations become naturalized, and their social production and historical specificity become obscured. Here I have posited that the genetic mapping of HIV has followed a similar cartographic trajectory: the drugs built to fight the virus and the tools built to study it are based on a very partial and contingent map of the virus, yet this map is rarely questioned or historicized.

Thus, not only is bioscientific knowledge about HIV in Africa limited, but most of the knowledge that does exist has been gleaned using tools predicated upon molecular maps of an HIV strain rarely found in Africa. It is *within* these tools that the geographic and economic inequalities of the

global epidemic have become embedded at the molecular level, in technologies that *always* refer back to wealthy countries in the global North—
Northern viruses, Northern research capacity, and Northern markets.
Whether or not these tools are able to accurately monitor non-B ("African")
viruses in clinical terms is a question that scientists are actively grappling
with. Ultimately, my argument is that regardless of the scientific outcomes,
it is politically urgent to juxtapose the willingness with which experts have
made very consequential knowledge claims about HIV in Africa—and particularly HIV drug resistance—with the near total absence of empirical research on the topic.

In this juxtaposition, we can see how the simultaneous deployment and
erasure of African bodies worked to support the claims of treatment skeptics. One the one hand, skeptics' fears regarding "antiretroviral anarchy"
and "doomsday strains" of drug-resistant HIV gained purchase from the
long tradition in Western discourse of framing an imagined "Africa" and
African bodies as outside the modern. On the other hand, the absence of
actual African bodies from the scientific study of HIV treatment and drug
resistance created a void of information into which these discourses could
easily step unchallenged. The positioning of African HIV subtypes as the
exceptions—the different or deviant viruses—and the Euro-American subtype as the universal standard fits what anthropologist Stacy Pigg has called
"the definition of marginality: to be positioned as the exception, the deviate,
the parochial, or the merely local in the face of the universal" (Pigg 2001,
510). For this reason, a key question for social and clinical scientists is not
only "What do we know about HIV in Africa?" but *"How* do we know
what we know?"

Chapter 3

The Turn toward Africa

"Africa is in vogue now," Dr. Jason Beale told me in early 2005. "Three or four years ago, no one would mention it." His comment was not intended to be flip. Rather, it was a joking acknowledgement of the way in which science is subject to its own form of trendiness that governs both interest in and funding of research projects. Beale is a warm and enthusiastic man, prone to mild exaggeration when trying to make a point, but earnest and persuasive nonetheless. He is both extremely ambitious and morally driven—a combination that has served him well in advancing his HIV research, first in the United States, and then in Uganda. To prove his point about the research trend, he urged me to search the abstracts of the last several years of the Conference on Retroviruses and Opportunistic Infections—the United States' most prestigious scientific AIDS conference—for the word "Africa." "It probably won't even be mentioned until 2002 or 2003," he told me. Beale's prediction proved to be generally true, if somewhat overstated. A search of the abstracts for "Africa" showed a steady increase between 1997 and 2006, ranging from a low of six in 1998 to a high of ninety-one in 2005.[1] This trend would continue in the years to follow. By 2011, the number of conference abstracts referencing "Africa" had risen to 174.

Dr. Beale was himself new to research in Africa. An HIV doctor turned researcher at the University of California, Beale focused his scientific career around the study of access and adherence to HIV medications among the poor and disadvantaged. His early work among urban homeless populations in the United States, described in chapter 1, made the case for universal HIV treatment access by demonstrating that even the most impoverished and socially marginalized patients were capable of taking complex drug regimens successfully. In the early 2000s, Beale began to shift his research focus to HIV treatment in Africa. As they had in their U.S. research, Beale and his colleagues sought to study patient drug-taking empirically, this time setting up shop in Kampala, the capital city of Uganda, a country known for its friendliness toward foreign researchers and its successful HIV prevention efforts (Thornton 2008). A few years later, when Kampala started to grow crowded with international researchers, he relocated his work to the town of Mbarara, four and a half hours away in rural western Uganda. At the time that Beale began working in Uganda, the free antiretroviral programs initiated by the Global Fund and PEPFAR were still several years away, but access to ARVs was slowly improving with the importation of cheaper generic ARVs from India. Beale's studies initially followed patients who were buying generic drugs out of pocket, and later included those who received free ARVs through the international programs.[2]

In this chapter, I use the stories of Dr. Beale and other American researchers to track what I call the "turn toward Africa" in U.S. HIV medicine. Dr. Beale, like many of his colleagues, expanded his research from one epicenter of the epidemic (the San Francisco Bay Area) to another one (East Africa) as HIV deaths stabilized in the United States and the push for treatment access in Africa gained political traction. I argue that this

---

1. Abstracts and keywords were searched using the "search abstracts" feature on the conference website. Because abstracts containing the phrase "African American" also appeared when searching under "Africa," I conducted searches under both terms and then subtracted the abstracts referring to African Americans from the total. While not an exact measure, this method gives a rough sense of how many papers were using data collected on the African continent. The earliest year for which abstracts were available on line was 1997.

2. In other words, patients enrolled in the studies obtained antiretrovirals on their own, not through Beale's research.

shift necessitated the translation of HIV disease from the qualitative, clinical language that predominates in Uganda into the quantitative, molecular terms deemed legitimate by U.S. doctors, medical journals, and funding bodies. This chapter shows how the ability to perform this kind of translation necessitates a certain kind of laboratory, and how access to such facilities can play a powerful role in governing who is able to participate in the making of global health science.

While the laboratory's importance in conferring scientific legitimacy has been well documented by science studies scholars, in low-income, postcolonial settings, laboratories wield an additional power to include or exclude scientists from the global South from participation in international science. This is another side of the molecular politics of global health described in the previous chapter. Aspiring African researchers have access to a surfeit of HIV patients from which to generate knowledge about the epidemic. (Indeed, it is this wealth of patients that draws American and other foreign HIV researchers to the continent.) However, they often lack the facilities necessary to conduct even the most basic molecular measurements, such as CD4 counts and viral load assessments, needed to make their studies publishable in major medical journals. Thus, in low-income African countries, the ability to participate as an equal in the international scientific arena often rests on access to elite, donor-funded laboratories. It is these "state-of-the-art" facilities that can provide the tools necessary to translate the often overwhelming level of clinical suffering in African clinics and public hospitals into terms considered scientifically legitimate in the global North. This suggests that the molecular terms of "global" health science are actually set *locally*, in the United States, Europe, and other technologically rich parts of the world, where the rise of randomized controlled trials and evidence-based medicine have rendered the clinic and the laboratory increasingly inseparable (Löwy 2000; Adams 2010b).

Golden Opportunities

Dr. Beale and other U.S. researchers were drawn to studying HIV in Africa by both humanitarian sentiment and scientific ambition. Having witnessed the seemingly miraculous impact of antiretrovirals on their own patients, American physician-researchers like Beale felt a moral imperative to use their expertise to address the increasingly destructive epidemic in Africa. In addition, American HIV scientists saw a unique opportunity in Africa's untreated epidemic. By the early 2000s, efforts to garner international support for free ARV medications in Africa had turned a corner. The Global Fund to Fight AIDS, Tuberculosis, and Malaria was founded in 2001, and less than two years later PEPFAR was announced. Moreover, on World AIDS Day in 2003, the WHO and UNAIDS launched their 3x5 Initiative, which advocated a target of treating three million people in low-income countries with ARVs by the end of the year 2005.[3] It would take several years for these programs to actually materialize on the ground and succeed in getting "drugs into bodies." For U.S. HIV researchers, the prospect of large numbers of African patients on the cusp of receiving their first antiretroviral medications presented a scientific opportunity that could not be found domestically. Thus, researchers' humanitarian motivations to work in Africa were paired with scientific ambitions aimed at taking advantage of the valuable research opportunity that African countries were seen as offering at the time.

A vignette from my participant-observation among a team of American epidemiologists illustrates the importance of Africa as a research opportunity to Beale and his colleagues. In February of 2005, I sat in on a meeting attended by eight health researchers at the University of California, San Francisco (UCSF). Their agenda was to design a research protocol that could be used across the university's growing number of HIV studies being conducted in Africa. They needed to develop a standardized way of collecting social, behavioral, and biological information from African HIV patients participating in research so that the data could then be "pooled" across studies conducted in different countries, in order to create larger and more powerful data sets for researchers to work with. Data regarding the advent of antiretroviral treatment in Africa was of particular interest because it provided a second chance to study the impact of HIV drugs on a large population of previously untreated people—a research opportunity that had been, in the words of the meeting's organizer, "lost" in the United States. As the group discussed how large a blood sample would be necessary

---

3. The 3x5 Initiative promoted expanded antiretroviral access but did not actually provide funding for treatment. The target of three million was met, but not until 2007.

in order to obtain the desired biological data, the researcher leading the meeting suggested that the African study participants have their blood drawn twice, arguing, "I can't emphasize this enough—a biological specimen in the pre-treatment era is just golden to us. And 7mls of blood just isn't enough."

Afterwards I asked Dr. Beale what the meeting's organizer had meant when he said a research opportunity had been "lost" in the United States. What Africa now offered, Beale told me, was the possibility of studying the virus as it evolved in relation to exposure to drugs. The UCSF researchers believed that knowledge about this evolution could provide useful information about both the pathophysiology and treatment of HIV. The opportunity to conduct such a study had been lost in the United States because effective drugs became available here much earlier in the epidemic, before researchers realized what Beale called the "scientific value" of such a project. This recognition of scientific value would come later, after the development of viral load and drug-resistance tests that allowed researchers to study the impact of antiretroviral drugs at the molecular level, rather than simply at the level of the patient's body (the clinical level). As a result, researchers did not begin to study the impact of treatment in this way until after drugs had been available for several years, by which time most U.S. patients had already been exposed to HIV medications and were likely to harbor drug-resistance mutations. They were no longer the pharmacological blank slates preferred by researchers. Thus, the opportunity to study the impact of HIV drugs on a large number of previously untreated (or "treatment-naïve") patients in the United States was seen as "lost." This was precisely the opportunity that Africa now offered.

In Kampala, Ugandan researchers were well aware of these opportunities. As I described in the introduction to this book, Kampala's Makerere University Medical School and its affiliated teaching hospital were premiere institutions of medical research in East Africa until the 1970s, when the dictatorship of Idi Amin devastated both their physical infrastructure and faculty (Iliffe 2002). During the rebuilding of Ugandan society during the 1980s, Makerere researchers conducted some of the earliest published research on AIDS in Africa in collaboration with international colleagues. With little domestic government money available for research, these scientists welcomed foreign interest in their epidemic as a means by which to obtain funding for their own research endeavors and careers. They understood that their large pool of patients was an asset that could not be found elsewhere. Dr. Joseph Muhwezi, a Makerere professor of pediatric infectious disease whom I interviewed in 2005, was particularly eloquent on this point. Muhwezi is an outspoken member of Makerere's scientific elite and the founder of a regional medical journal aimed at providing researchers an African-run venue for publishing their work. Reflecting on his own collaborations with European researchers, he made the following case for Uganda as a fertile environment for knowledge production:

> Yes, we want the state of the art, but what does the state of the art mean? For me, the state of the art means finding your niche where you are best and excelling in it. So if you want [to learn about] clinical care of HIV-infected children, the place to go is Uganda. If I go to the Netherlands, they don't even have patients. There's not even one child with HIV anymore in the Netherlands. There's not even one child! That's where we excel. We have clinical patients. We have loads and loads of patients. Other people don't have patients! They are training doctors under video—I saw it in the Netherlands. They have never touched patients! What type doctors are you going to produce? You work for us, our doctors, if there is an operation, the students go there. And they feel, they assist, they touch. And that's the excellence we want. Molecules and things, they are very important, but at the end of the day—it's the person that matters, in my view.

Importantly, Muhwezi's acknowledgement of opportunity has embedded within it an assertion of "excellence," or expertise—specifically, clinical expertise—as well as a value judgment that clinical expertise is ultimately more important than knowledge dependent upon technology.

During the course of my fieldwork, I encountered a number of physician-researchers from the United States and other countries in the global North who expressed admiration for the hands-on clinical acumen and flexibility wielded by their Ugandan colleagues. They were impressed by the ability of Ugandan clinicians to practice medicine without many of the basic medications and technologies Northern doctors had become dependent upon.[4] Yet they often paired this respect for the Ugandans' skills with uneasiness about

---

4. See Wendland 2010 (chapter 6) for the perspectives of Malawian doctors on their own clinical expertise and creative ingenuity in the context of scarcity.

the accuracy of diagnosis based on clinical symptoms. For example, while conducting research in Kampala in 2005 I met George Avery, a Canadian doctor teaching in an HIV-medicine training program based at Makerere Medical School's Infectious Disease Institute. During the daily "tea break" between morning lectures, I asked him to reflect on the low-tech environment in which most of the African trainees were working. As we snacked on hot tea, samosas, and boiled eggs that had been brought up for the class from the canteen, he told me that the African clinicians had very good clinical skills "because they don't have the diagnostics to fall back on the way Western doctors do." Then he told me the story of a Ugandan doctor he had observed evaluating a patient. The doctor's clinical examination suggested one diagnosis but the chest x-ray suggested another, and he had told his colleagues that he wasn't sure which he should trust. "In the West," Dr. Avery continued, "there would be no question—you would go with the x-ray." But in Uganda, he said, doctors are so confident in their clinical findings that it can actually lead them to doubt the diagnostics. He told this story with both a sense of awe for the clinical skills of the Ugandan physician, but also a sense of disbelief and discomfort with questioning the x-ray's results.

For international researchers, Uganda's clinics presented both an opportunity and a challenge. As Dr. Muhwezi notes, Uganda's patient-rich but "resource-poor" environment offered a chance for learning that could not be matched in wealthier, healthier countries. As I describe in chapter 5, this is an opportunity well known to visiting American medical students, who often find they are allowed much greater access to the bodies of African patients than they have to patients' bodies back home. However, clinical expertise is less valuable in the world of international research, which answers to the standards set by leading journals and funding bodies. Because these journals and funders are located almost exclusively in the United States and Europe, their standards reflect the highly technologically mediated and increasingly molecularized "evidence-based" medicine that is upheld as state of the art in these parts of the world (Adams 2010b). In this "global" scientific arena, researchers are expected to produce data that is both quantifiable and *portable*—in other words, data that can circulate internationally and be compared to data collected elsewhere (Petryna 2009). This is what the UCSF researchers were after in designing a common research protocol that could be used across the university's various studies on the African continent. It is also what Dr. Beale needed in order to generate Ugandan data that was commensurable with existing data on HIV treatment collected in the United States. In other words, in the transnational research arena, Dr. Muhwezi's assertion that "at the end of the day—it's the person that matters" more than "molecules and things," does not really hold. In global health science, it is "molecules and things," not clinical signs and symptoms, that most often bear the mark of scientific legitimacy. However advanced the clinical skills of Ugandan physician-researchers might be, this expertise is of little value in the world of global science, where it is viewed as qualitative and localized rather than quantitative and generalizable (Adams 2010a; Feierman 2011).

Thus, for Beale and other U.S. researchers shifting their research toward Africa, a key step in generating authoritative scientific findings would be translating the clinical epidemic they confronted in "resource-poor" African clinics and hospitals into the molecular terms that would render it commensurable with data collected in "resource-rich" parts of the world. The encounter between their highly technical understanding of HIV and the clinical spectacle of human suffering they were to encounter in African hospitals was one they would find at once scientifically challenging, emotionally draining, and oddly nostalgic.

Clinical Nostalgia

Dr. Beale had never traveled to Africa until he began planning a research project in Uganda. This was not unusual among the American researchers I spoke with over the course of my fieldwork, and applied to myself as well. For him and for other American physician-scientists who had treated patients in the early days of the U.S. epidemic, the first trip to Uganda was often a confrontation with striking familiarity embedded in a context of profound difference. These differences ranged from the ordinary variation in language (though many Ugandans speak English), landscape, and culture encountered when traveling to any foreign country, to much starker contrasts of race and wealth. For example, "whiteness" was no longer the unmarked category it so often is in the United States; instead, white skin was highly conspicuous in an overwhelmingly black- and brown-skinned nation, and *muzungu*—the Luganda term[5] for foreigner or white person—was often the first local vocabulary that the predominantly white American researchers learned. This difference was further accentuated by the contrast between Uganda's poverty and America's wealth, and the realization that elements of daily living often taken for granted in the United States—such as electricity, public transit, ATM machines,[6] residential street addresses, and refrigeration—were suddenly unreliable, confusing, or not available. The reliance on a cash-based economy and the rarity of receipts was particularly vexing for Beale's grant manager at the University of California, who was constantly struggling to produce a paper trail showing how the project's funds were being spent in Uganda.

American researchers turning their attention to Africa were confronted with the social and logistical realities of what it means to conduct research in a "resource-poor country" or a "resource-limited setting"—the terms most commonly used in international HIV research to describe low-income countries like Uganda. Dr. Beale, having spent years working in New York and San Francisco's poorest county hospitals, was no stranger to poverty and inequality. However, the signs of this poverty—young boys with bathroom scales selling passersby the opportunity to weigh themselves, women scavenging for wood to turn into charcoal they could sell, and the coffin shops lining the road between the airport and the capital city—were radically different from the urban poverty he was accustomed to in his "resource-rich" country. This confrontation with difference went both ways: when Beale's Ugandan staff began visiting San Francisco, they were deeply shocked by the large numbers of homeless people living and sleeping on the downtown streets, a rare sight in Uganda.

Yet, within this world of difference, visiting American researchers encountered an eerie familiarity upon entering the inpatient wards of

---

5. Luganda is one of the approximately forty African languages spoken in Uganda, and is the dominant local language in the capital city and surrounding areas. *Muzungu* is a word used for foreigner or "white person" in many East African Bantu languages, including Swahili (*mzungu*). English is Uganda's national language, a legacy of British colonialism, and is widely spoken among the educated classes.

6. The first time I traveled to Uganda, in 2003, ATM machines were not available and I had to arrive with enough money in cash and travelers' checks to cover two months of living expenses. By 2005, cash machines were common in downtown Kampala, and by 2009 they were also present in Mbarara.

Kampala's hospitals, where they saw patients with AIDS dying from infections they had not encountered since the first days of the U.S. epidemic. The experience was particularly striking, Dr. Beale told me, for those coming from the San Francisco area—a city that had been emblematic of the epidemic in the United States in the early 1980s much the same way that Uganda was to become emblematic of AIDS in Africa in the early 1990s. He described a senior colleague as getting "almost wistful" or "nostalgic" in Uganda's hospitals because he was reminded of his experience working in San Francisco General Hospital in the 1980s. He also told me of a young, gay epidemiologist on his staff who began crying when he first walked through the inpatient wards in Kampala because it reminded him of the partner he had lost to AIDS, of his friends who had died, and of what Beale described as the "slaughter" that was San Francisco before the discovery of effective HIV drugs.

The Bay Area–based AIDS researchers that I followed to Uganda often described the epidemic they saw there as resembling San Francisco in the pre-treatment era. They gave this description both with horror over the extreme and unnecessary suffering caused by the lack of drugs, and with the "nostalgia" that Dr. Beale identified. For Beale himself, this nostalgia was for a time when he felt he was really a part of a team, fighting a disease that no one understood, and caring for patients who had become social and medical pariahs in much of the rest of the country. The nostalgia was not about wishing the drugs did not exist—on the contrary, he has heavily advocated for expanded access to treatment throughout his career. Rather, it was about the kind of doctor he had been able to be in that era. "Right now," he told me in 2005, "HIV medicine is much more technical and much less human" than it used to be:

> In the 1980s, it was all human, because comfort and care were the only and the best thing you could provide. It was horrific, but it was also terrific because the staff was so close, and so dedicated. It was a very special relationship. Now, HIV medicine in the U.S. is much more frightening. It used to be about providing a painless and meaningful death. Now a death is a mistake. The cost of making an error is much higher, because the standard is that everyone lives. Now, making a technical error could have a major impact on patient survival. The weight of technical errors is much heavier now [when there are twenty drugs available] than in the '80s and early '90s, when there

were only one to four drugs and none of them worked very well. Then there were fewer mistakes to be made, and mistakes didn't impact the outcome anyway. In the 1980s, the human was the best you had.[7]

Yet it would be a gross oversimplification to say that AIDS in Uganda is simply a time-delayed version of what AIDS was in San Francisco. Despite any nostalgia that they may have felt, when American AIDS doctors began traveling to Uganda and other African countries experiencing serious HIV epidemics, they encountered a disease that was fundamentally different in many ways than AIDS as they knew it, despite its eerie familiarity. While some of the visible manifestations of untreated HIV disease may have reminded them of their own patients in the past (the Kaposi's sarcoma, the wasting syndrome, the cryptococcal meningitis), other elements suggested an epidemic that is not commensurable with AIDS in the United States: the background of endemic malaria and malnutrition against which the infection plays out, additional "tropical" diseases not seen in the United States, and the large numbers of women and children with HIV. There were less visible differences, too, such as the distinct HIV subtypes described in the previous chapter.

The experiences of another Bay Area doctor highlight this tension between familiarity and difference that characterizes the turn toward Africa in American AIDS research. I met with Dr. Richard Swan in his office in downtown San Francisco in 2005. At the time, he was the director of a global HIV/AIDS foundation that supported HIV clinics and treatment in Africa, China, and the Caribbean. He had first encountered AIDS when working as a doctor at San Francisco General, the county's public hospital, when the epidemic hit in the early 1980s. In the 1990s he switched his focus to health policy and became a prominent member of the Clinton administration and an advocate for greater attention to the impact of AIDS on

---

7. Claire Wendland describes similar feelings of shared humanity among present-day Malawian physicians and medical students, and links these feelings to the low-technology, high-risk conditions in which they must practice. "Not insulated from suffering by technology or equipment, or private patient rooms with walls and curtains, or high staffing levels that allowed nurses to do all the dirty work, or vaccines or postexposure prophylaxis that limited their risks of contracting killer diseases when they stuck themselves with bloody needles, these student doctors were made constantly aware that they were, as [medical student] Zaithwa Mthindi said, 'as human as everybody else'" (Wendland 2010, 180).

African American communities. (Years after our interview, he would even-tually return to Washington to assume a leadership role in the PEPFAR program.) While working for the federal government in the late 1990s he served as a representative to UNAIDS, the United Nations body dealing with the global AIDS epidemic. The UNAIDS meetings were often held in areas of the world heavily affected by HIV, and in traveling to these places Dr. Swan found himself immersed in an epidemic that reminded him of his early days at San Francisco General Hospital, yet far exceeding anything he had witnessed in the United States. His reflections on this time are worth quoting at length:

> My travel in the developing world started around 1995 or 1996. I had to go to these quarterly meetings of UNAIDS, which would be held in Lusaka in Zambia, in Khayelitsha in South Africa, in Durban in South Africa, in Zim-babwe. They put them in areas that were heavily impacted by HIV. And so through the course of that, I began to see all of these extraordinary things.
>
> For a clinician to walk into hospital after hospital where people are standing in the hallways, they're sleeping in the hallways, they're two people in the bed, one underneath the bed—you have these large, open wards. I can remember being in Zambia about two hours outside of Lusaka, and we had been taken to this Salvation Army hospital that truly was out in nowhere, that was big—and in a ward of about sixty beds times three [three times as many patients as beds], there were probably twenty people with grand mal seizures, seizing in the beds, just from untreated cryptococcal meningitis. And the standard of care there—this was '98 or maybe '97—drugs that we all knew how to use were not available. Diflucan [fluconazole] was out; am-photericin, which is the drug of choice [for cryptococcal meningitis] was ab-solutely available but [they] couldn't pay for it. It was really startling, and that was when my mind started to say, "The need that I'm seeing is extraordi-nary, and it's completely unmet and unaddressed." And I began to think about the ethics of ignoring it, and not being able to ignore it.
>
> . . . So I started realizing that the epidemic really wasn't happening in North America at all, and was happening elsewhere. And not only that, having been a pre-ARV clinician [in the United States], I realized that all of what I knew was directly applicable to what I was seeing. These were people who've never seen ARVs. These are people who are dealing with opportu-nistic infections, and that's what we did up until 1994, in the United States. Fifty percent of the gay men in San Francisco were infected when I was in San Francisco. We were *full* on the in-patient service at San Francisco General

Hospital; 70 to 80 percent of the patients in the hospital, all services, were AIDS-related. The emergency room was full of people coming in with complaints of infections related to HIV.

While Swan never uses the word "nostalgia" to describe his experiences in Africa, what he saw in Zambia in the 1990s clearly brought back memories of working in San Francisco in the 1980s. Swan's description of the crowded hospital and lack of medications in Zambia flows directly into his reminiscence of San Francisco General Hospital prior to the discovery of effective HIV medications in 1995. As a clinician, he realized that having worked in the pre-treatment era in the United States gave him experience treating the kinds of infections he was now witnessing in Africa. This eerie kinship between AIDS in San Francisco in the 1980s and AIDS in Africa in the 1990s and 2000s means that American doctors like Beale and Swan experienced their early trips to Africa as "travel across both place and time, not just to far away, but to long ago" (Wendland 2012, 116; see also Brada 2011b).

Yet, this clinical familiarity was paired with differences in scale and economics that were shocking to a doctor accustomed to the health care system of a wealthy nation. This is evident in Swan's description of the Zambian Salvation Army hospital—the open wards crowded to three times their capacity, two patients to each bed and a third on the floor, the simultaneous seizures among twenty patients from untreated meningitis—in which the epidemic takes on a spectacular level of suffering unmatched at even the most impacted hospitals in the United States in the 1980s. This is the dark side of the much more "human" and much less "technical" pre-ARV HIV medicine described by Dr. Beale; the "horrific" counterpoint to the "terrific" feeling of staff bonding and medical mission that the pre-treatment era fostered for San Francisco AIDS doctors.

AIDS by the Numbers

Uncertainty about the nature of AIDS and conjecture that it might be different in Africa than in the United States and Europe has existed since the early years of the epidemic. In 1985 *The Lancet* published an article by Ugandan researchers working in the Rakai district near Uganda's southwestern border with Tanzania. The article described a "new disease" that people in Rakai were calling "slim" because of the severe weight loss it brought on. The authors claimed, "although slim disease resembles AIDS in many ways, it seems to be a new entity." The basis of their argument was that slim and AIDS looked different clinically and epidemiologically: AIDS was found mainly in "Western homosexual patients" whose chief symptoms were often Kaposi's sarcoma and swollen lymph nodes (lymphadenopathy). Slim, in contrast, was found "primarily in the heterosexually promiscuous popu-lation," and had diarrhea and severe weight loss as its primary markers (Serwadda et al. 1985). Within months the *Lancet* article's claim that slim was "new" was contested, as it became apparent that many Ugandans with slim did indeed suffer from Kaposi's sarcoma, and many Westerners with AIDS developed severe wasting, making AIDS and slim more similar than different. However, for a time, a tacit acknowledgement of difference per-sisted in the medical literature—the equation of "slim" with "AIDS" was initially qualified by a reference to Africa: slim was "identical" not to AIDS but to "African AIDS" or to "AIDS as seen in Africa" (Kamradt, Niese, and Vogel 1985).

Although the idea that slim and AIDS were different diseases was short-lived, it is nonetheless an instructive example of the difficulty of establishing a universal definition of a syndrome made up of an assortment of diseases whose manifestation varies across geography and patient populations. It also challenges the universality of disease categories, and aptly demonstrates the "local biologies" that emerge when biological and social processes inter-twine (Lock 1995; Lock and Nguyen 2010). Furthermore, the scientific sidelining of slim shows how Euro-American definitions of what constitutes "AIDS" have dominated the field from the very beginning. The vast major-ity of published papers describing AIDS at this time were based on research conducted among gay men in the United States and Europe. Thus, "AIDS" with no qualifier implied Euro-American AIDS, and this was the refer-ence point against which other (qualified or marked) manifestations of the disease—such as "African AIDS"—were compared.

These qualifiers are now less common in the medical literature, but questions of difference persist in global HIV medicine. AIDS does look different in different places, both in its epidemiology (who gets sick) and its pathophysiology (how they get sick). But in the current moment, perhaps the biggest difference between AIDS in the United States and AIDS in

Uganda is technological. Since the advent of effective antiretroviral drugs in 1995, HIV care in wealthy countries has grown increasingly molecularized. As Nikolas Rose has noted, this shift mirrors a more general trend toward the "molecular gaze" in biomedicine:

> The clinical gaze has been supplemented, if not supplanted, by this molecular gaze. . . . Life is now understood, and acted upon, at the molecular level, in terms of the functional properties of coding sequences of nucleotide bases and their variations, the molecular mechanisms that regulate expression and transcription, the link between the functional properties of proteins and their molecular topography, the formation of particular intracellular elements— ion channels, enzyme activities, transporter genes, membrane potentials— with their particular mechanical and biological properties. (Rose 2007, 12)

What Rose describes is a shift in scale: where clinical medicine works with the unit of the human body at the level of organs and vital systems (circulatory, respiratory, digestive, etc.), molecular medicine operates at the microscopic scale of the intracellular, the genomic, and the proteomic (protein manufacture).[8] Within HIV medicine, molecular technologies have had a huge impact and have yielded some of the most important therapeutic and diagnostic tools available to patients and their doctors. Protease inhibitors, the class of antiretroviral drugs that made the first successful triple-combination therapies possible, are the product of structure-based drug design, in which pharmaceuticals are engineered to interfere with viral replication at the molecular level. In addition, molecular diagnostic technologies that measure the strength of a patient's immune system (CD4 testing) and the level of virus in the blood (viral load) have taken on great importance in HIV care, and are now integral to treatment guidelines specifying when patients should be started on antiretrovirals. The same is true for HIV research, where these technologies provide a standardized means by which to track disease progression and treatment efficacy.

Molecular biology has shaped scientific responses to the AIDS epidemic since it first came into widespread public and scientific awareness in 1981.

---

8. As many scholars have noted, Rose's observations about the molecularization of medicine do not account for the sharp disparities in biomedical resources and practice across the globe, or what Matthew Sparke calls "the uneven global landscape of body counting" (Sparke 2013).

The isolation of the HIV virus in 1984 and the development of an effective HIV blood test shortly thereafter were both enabled by then-recent developments in molecular biology. As one historian noted in 1989, "From many points of view, the AIDS pandemic is necessarily a new disease; the pathology could not even exist as a concept before the recent discoveries made by molecular biology and immunology" (Fantini 1991, 53; see also Harden 1991). However, outside the laboratory, the molecularization of HIV medicine was a much more gradual process. For the first decade of the epidemic, an AIDS diagnosis in the United States (and elsewhere) was made according to clinical signs and symptoms, not the molecular diagnostics of CD4 cell count and viral load by which it is currently characterized. In 1982, shortly after the disease was named acquired immune deficiency syndrome, the CDC defined a case of AIDS as "a disease . . . occurring in a person with no known cause for diminished resistance to that disease. Such diseases include KS [Kaposi's sarcoma], PCP [Pneumocystis carinii pneumonia], and serious OOI [other opportunistic infections]" (CDC 1982). In the media and the public imagination, this definition of AIDS was embodied in images of gaunt young men covered with the iconic purple blotches of Kaposi's sarcoma.[9] In 1985, following the isolation of the HIV virus and development of a commercial blood test, the CDC added the criterion of a positive HIV blood test to the AIDS case definition, but otherwise this definition remained strictly symptom-based until 1993. Beginning in that year, the CDC expanded its definition of AIDS to include any individuals whose CD4 lymphocytes, or "helper T cells," had fallen below a count of 200 (CDC 1992).[10] Now there was a standardized, quantitative measure to define AIDS. Unlike Kaposi's, this measurement was also invisible, in that it was possible for a patient to have a CD4 count of less than 200 without having visible indicators of "full-blown AIDS."

CD4 cells or T cells are a key component of the body's immune system and a preferred target of the HIV virus, which kills them slowly over time,

---

9. Perhaps the best-known example of this is Alon Reininger's photograph of a dying San Francisco man titled "Ken Meeks, Patient With AIDS, Being Cared For By A Friend." It was named World Press Photo of the Year in 1986 and was published in *Life* magazine in 1988 (Museum of Contemporary Photography 2008).

10. A normal CD4 cell count ranges between about 500 to 1,500 cells per cubic millimeter of blood.

leaving the body increasingly vulnerable to disease. Low CD4 cell levels were documented in AIDS patients from the very beginning of the epidemic in 1981, and CD4 testing was used in the earliest U.S. effort to screen blood donations prior to the development of the HIV blood test (*The Lancet* 1981; Galel, Lifson, and Engleman 1995). The ability to measure CD4 levels was enabled by prior advances in molecular biology, principally the development of monoclonal antibody technology in 1975. Yet clinicians and researchers viewed CD4 testing as limited in its clinical and epidemiological utility, both because CD4 counts tend to be naturally changeable over time and because test results may vary across laboratories. This is perhaps why a measurement that is so integral to HIV medicine today was relatively marginal to AIDS care for the first twelve years of the epidemic.

This began to change with the 1993 inclusion of CD4 count within the CDC's official AIDS case definition. At the time, the decision to do so may have been largely political in nature. For years, the CDC had faced criticism that its list of AIDS-defining conditions was biased because it reflected the illnesses most commonly seen in gay men in the United States. (For example, gynecological conditions and "tropical" infections characteristic of AIDS in women or in the global South were not on the list). The addition of low CD4 count to the AIDS case definition was seen as a way to create objective disease criteria in response to these criticisms (Sheppard et al. 1993). In addition, CD4 testing was useful to researchers working to develop pharmaceuticals effective against HIV, as it provided a standardized numerical means by which to measure the impact of a drug on a patient's immune system (Schoenfeld, Finkelstein, and Richman 1993). The molecularization of HIV was furthered by the development of viral load testing in the mid-1990s, which used newly developed polymerase chain reaction technology to measure the concentration of virus circulating in a patient's blood, thus providing a quantitative method for measuring a drug's success in killing HIV (Löwy 2000). With the development and rapid dissemination of effective antiretroviral therapy in the United States in the mid- and late 1990s, CD4 and viral load testing became integrated into clinical care as quantitative methods for monitoring patient response to these powerful new medications. These tests, known in medicine as "surrogate markers," made it possible to respond to warning signs of declining health (such as a falling CD4 count or a spike in viral load) before a patient fell ill with potentially life-threatening opportunistic infections. Indeed, in the United

States, the technologies of CD4 count and viral load measurements are now inextricably bound to the way that HIV and AIDS are conceptualized, studied, and treated. As a result, in a U.S. context, it is nearly impossible to have a medical discussion about HIV without referring to CD4 count and viral load.

The situation in Uganda and other low-income countries is quite different. When Dr. Beale began conducting HIV research in Uganda in the early 2000s, patients could receive a blood test to detect HIV infection, but after testing positive patients' disease progression was measured largely according to clinical symptoms, since CD4 testing was possible only on a limited basis and only in Kampala. In the absence of molecular monitoring technologies, doctors used "clinical monitoring"—physical examination and bodily signs such as weight loss, hair texture, and skin condition—to assess their patients' proximity to an AIDS diagnosis. Ugandan physicians and researchers recorded patients' status using the World Health Organization's "staging" system for HIV. This system is a categorization of progression toward death based on weight loss and infections, in which Stage I represents asymptomatic HIV infection and Stage IV (the final stage) constitutes advanced, bedridden illness. Although the availability of CD4 testing in Ugandan clinics has grown significantly since PEPFAR and the Global Fund began providing free treatment in late 2004, access to more expensive viral load tests remains very limited and drug-resistance testing is extremely rare. Thus, clinical monitoring remains a principal means of determining the extent of a patient's HIV disease, and—for those able to access antiretroviral medications—of discerning whether or not the drugs are working.

"Clinical monitoring" is perhaps best explained as hands-on doctoring: assessing the patient's condition primarily through physical examination, supplemented by very basic laboratory tests when available. Doctors may feel the texture of a patient's hair, the condition of his or her skin, and the firmness of the abdomen and lymph nodes. They look for rashes, thrush, lesions, clubbing of the fingertips—all indicators of possible AIDS-related illnesses. They note whether their patient is losing weight or seems dehydrated, or if one side of the chest is rising more than the other when the patient breathes. And they listen very closely to the lungs for sounds that might warn of pneumonia or tuberculosis. One of the tricky aspects of managing HIV treatment in the absence of molecular monitoring technologies is that many of the side effects of antiretroviral medications closely resemble symptoms of AIDS-related illnesses. Diarrhea, changes in body fat (lipodystrophy), pain in the extremities (peripheral neuropathy), and rash are all potential antiretroviral side effects that can also be signs of AIDS. Thus, in the absence of lab work, Ugandan clinicians find following patients on antiretroviral therapy to be an exercise in uncertainty, in which the bodily manifestations of successful treatment can be difficult to distinguish from symptoms of the disease itself (see also Okeke 2011).

Giving Them a Laboratory

For American researchers like Beale, bridging the technological divide between HIV medicine in the United States and Uganda is a matter of professional scientific survival. While clinical monitoring is seen as an acceptable, if flawed, answer to the lack of laboratory monitoring technologies available to Ugandan doctors in the clinic, it is not an acceptable means of assessing HIV disease progression for the purposes of global health science. Without the molecular quantitative measures afforded by CD4, viral load, and drug-resistance testing, Beale's research would be essentially unfundable and unpublishable. Thus, his establishment of a successful research project in Uganda has been contingent upon his ability to translate the "molar" body of "limbs, organs, [and] tissues" found in the clinic to the "molecular" body that NIH grant applications and leading journals insist upon (Rose 2007, 11).

As Bruno Latour has famously described, laboratories are what make this kind of translation possible, because they transform the disorder of nature into orderly data, suitable for making persuasive scientific arguments (Latour and Woolgar 1979; Latour 1983, 1987, 1999). This is certainly the case for Dr. Beale and other American HIV researchers working in Uganda, who rely heavily upon the services of a few select laboratories in order to render the disease in the molecular terms required by their funders and publishers. However, what Latour's otherwise helpful insight leaves unconsidered are the power dynamics particular to labs in the postcolonial world, where in addition to being "centers of calculation," laboratories may also be donor-funded development projects, products of medical humanitarianism, or facilities built to enable the work of visiting and expatriate scientists. Often they are all three, as was the case with Beale's primary laboratory at Kampala's Infectious Diseases Institute (IDI), which was built in 2004.

The Institute was the brain child of Max Edwards, an American infectious disease doctor who, like many senior AIDS researchers in the United States, made a name for himself treating and researching AIDS in San Francisco during the first years of the epidemic. He began working in Uganda in 1989, as part of a U.S.-funded study of heterosexual transmission of HIV. In addition to his career in academia, Dr. Edwards spent seventeen years as a member of the scientific advisory board of Pfizer, one of the most profitable pharmaceutical manufacturers in the world. Edwards, who died in 2007, was notorious among his university colleagues for his sociability and powers of persuasion. Thus it was not as surprising as it might have been when, over dinner in 2001, he managed to parlay his friendship with the CEO of Pfizer into a $5 million grant from the company's philanthropic foundation to support the building of the IDI. In addition to providing spaces for clinical care and physician-training programs, the IDI would also include a state-of-the-art research laboratory. The Institute would be affiliated with Makerere University's medical school and be located on the campus of Mulago Hospital, the university's teaching facility, where its new construction and bright exterior made it stand out against the sooty, weathered façade of the adjacent main hospital building—an architectural testament to the special access to donor money that HIV holds over other afflictions.

Upon its completion in 2004, the building was christened with a gala grand opening celebration presided over by Ugandan President Yoweri Museveni. The guests at the celebration represented the numerous stakeholders in the Institute and illustrated the complex web of alliances and jockeying for power that has characterized the Institute's administration. In addition to President Museveni and the Pfizer CEO, the dedication was attended by members of the Academic Alliance, a collaboration of U.S. and Ugandan HIV physician-researchers organized by Max Edwards to govern the institute and raise funds for its continued support. Two other groups of American stakeholders also participated in the grand opening: U.S. HIV researchers who had ongoing studies based at Makerere Medical School, and representatives of Richard Swan's San Francisco–based foundation, which was the fiscal agent for Pfizer's donation and had overseen the construction of the Institute.

The rationale for building the IDI varies according to the accounts of different stakeholders, as do feelings about its appropriateness. In interviews with me, its boosters described the Institute as a way to leave something tangible to benefit Makerere Medical School and Mulago Hospital, repeatedly pointing out that it was the first building to be built on the teaching hospital's campus in thirty-seven years. It is also true, of course, that the building provides a very visible example of Pfizer's corporate philanthropy, one that helps the company promote itself as being in the business of saving lives in Africa even as it defends the drug-patenting laws that put medicines financially out of reach for many in Uganda (Milford 2011). Publicly, the Institute's training program for African doctors has been promoted as the Institute's primary raison d'etre, and Max Edwards echoed this sentiment in his interview with me. Privately, some stakeholders—including Richard Swan and a few North American researchers—suggested to me that the IDI's state-of-the-art, U.S.-certified laboratory was actually the jewel in the crown, built to attract more internationally funded research projects and to benefit the research of North American members of the Academic Alliance. Indeed, the IDI became a lynchpin of international HIV research in Uganda almost instantly upon opening its doors. During my fieldwork there in 2005, moped couriers from the global shipping service DHL regularly visited the building, testifying to the constant transnational flow of materials and information circulating through the institute.

The facility's power to attract high-profile American AIDS researchers was made clear to me by Karl da Silva, a colleague of Beale's and the director of a prominent, nonprofit California virology research center. In his San Francisco laboratory, Da Silva was spearheading what was viewed as some of the most exciting and promising research on the molecular biology of HIV—research that could lead to entirely new ways of treating the disease. At the time of our interview in late 2004, his virology center had just moved into a gleaming new building in a formerly industrial part of the city that was then being redeveloped into a biotechnology research campus. His office offered an expansive view of the surrounding area and the assortment of corporate and university research facilities being built through the city's public-private redevelopment initiative.

Da Silva was avuncular in manner and enthusiastic yet humble about his own research. He had just returned from Kampala, where he had attended the dedication ceremony for the IDI building at the invitation of American colleagues involved with the Institute. It had been his first trip to Africa, and he spoke like a converted man, decrying the lack of adequate medical treatment, the underequipped hospital, and an average life span nearly cut in half by AIDS. "The scope of the problem," he told me, "is *immense*." As a result of his trip, he said, he was determined to start a research project of his own in Uganda. The new laboratory housed within the Institute made this determination possible. Though it was not the only high-quality research lab in Kampala, the researchers I spoke with regarded it as the best. I was told several times that it was the only laboratory in East Africa to be certified by the College of American Pathologists.[11] This certification meant that the tests conducted there were quality controlled, audited on a regular basis, and acceptable for clinical trials and the registration of new drugs. As such, it was preferred by major funding agencies such as the NIH and its British equivalent, the Medical Research Council, as well as by drug companies.

For Da Silva, the lab made it possible to carry out biological analyses in Kampala, rather than dealing with the complicated shipment of perishable biological materials across several continents to a U.S. lab:

> It becomes a bit problematic to be trying to send cells from Uganda to here [California]. A lot of times they get stuck in customs in some country or they get lost. Or they thaw, and valuable samples are lost. The IDI offers the opportunity to actually be able to do a lot of the analysis right there, from fresh samples, which is far better.

Like Da Silva, Dr. Beale was initially attracted to the IDI lab because of its sophisticated technology and reputation for excellence. (In addition, both researchers were former colleagues of Max Edwards, who earlier in his career had treated patients at San Francisco General Hospital and founded the virology institute that Da Silva would later head). Furthermore, during his first years working in Uganda—when his research was still based in

---

11. This was the case until an additional U.S.-supported laboratory was certified at Makerere in July 2005. This was followed by certification of a lab in Tanzania in 2007, one in Kenya in 2009, and a third lab in Uganda in 2009. All three currently certified Ugandan labs are in or near the capital city of Kampala, and all receive support from U.S. universities or government agencies (College of American Pathologists 2012).

Kampala—Beale found the lab's central location convenient, much as Da Silva did. However, even after moving his research several hours away to Mbarara, Beale continued to use the IDI as his primary laboratory facility. His allegiance to the Kampala lab, and the considerable logistical challenges he was willing to overcome in order to continue to have his samples processed there, speaks to the power of a U.S.-sanctioned laboratory in postcolonial science. It also speaks to an evolving geography of scientific inclusion and exclusion within Uganda.

Geographies of Power

Dr. Beale's decision to relocate his research to Mbarara was in part intended to counter critiques that his Kampala findings were not representative of Uganda's primarily agrarian population. Although Mbarara town is relatively urban by Ugandan standards, the Wellness Clinic from which Beale would enroll his study participants drew patients from a wide swath of surrounding rural areas. Many patients supported themselves through small-scale farming or gardening, and some traveled long distances on public transit to make their monthly clinic visits. In addition, Beale found that Kampala had grown crowded with international researchers attracted to the safe and friendly English-speaking city and its internationally known medical school. Prominent Ugandan researchers at Makerere found themselves increasingly bombarded with requests to collaborate as competition for research sites and subjects in Kampala grew. This meant that Beale and other researchers now had to put more and more energy into competing with each other for relationships with Ugandan researchers and their patients. Even though it was home to a university, Mbarara was off the beaten track for foreign medical researchers. The Mbarara University of Science and Technology and the Wellness Clinic welcomed Beale's University of California team as their first major international research collaborators.

The scientific value of Beale's relocation to Mbarara derived from the town's comparatively remote geographic location, which researchers from the United States and Europe perceived as a more authentic representation of Uganda—and even Africa as a whole—than Kampala's urban environment. This was brought home to me in 2005, when I trailed a pair of visiting Swiss researchers as they toured the wards of Mbarara's teaching hospital.

The Swiss were in Mbarara at Beale's invitation, and he was courting them as potential research collaborators. Their research involved the comparison of patients' biological responses to ARV treatment in Africa to those in wealthy parts of the world, in hopes of providing scientific evidence that Africans were benefiting from the treatment as much as Americans and Europeans had. Though they deplored the unequal health care conditions suffered by African HIV doctors and patients, they nonetheless observed the crumbling buildings, rusting bed frames, and crowded conditions of Mbarara's hospital with a form of approval, assuring each other that Mbarara had "real wards," unlike the well-appointed, corporate-funded outpatient clinic at the IDI in Kampala.

For Beale, the scientific legitimacy gained by working in the more "authentic" environment of Mbarara had to be balanced against the scientific risk posed by the area's lack of trustworthy laboratory infrastructure. For this reason, Beale decided to continue to use the IDI lab in Kampala rather than process his blood samples locally. At the time he began his research, little could be done with the samples in Mbarara. The Wellness Clinic's sole CD4 machine was notoriously slow and unreliable, and viral load testing was completely unavailable. In addition, Beale needed a facility that could reliably store and ship some of his samples back to the United States, as certain tests necessary for his research (such as drug-resistance genotyping) were not available in Uganda. Again, these storage and shipping services were not available in Mbarara. Lastly, the IDI's certification by the College of American Pathologists ensured quality results that would be accepted as commensurable with results derived from a U.S. laboratory.

In order to continue using the IDI lab, Beale's research team went through considerable trouble to transport the blood samples taken from patients in Mbarara to the laboratory in Kampala in a timely manner. The route was about four hours (and sometimes five, with road work) on a two-lane paved road through rolling countryside punctuated by small roadside trading stops, family farm plots and grazing lands, and an occasional large town. Samples needed to be delivered to the laboratory on the same day they were drawn in order to prevent them from deteriorating. This meant scheduling all patient blood draws in Mbarara between 7:00 and 10:00 am so that the samples could arrive in Kampala by mid-afternoon, when the IDI lab closed. It also necessitated finding a reliable and affordable way to transport the samples to the capital city on a daily basis. This task was left up to Eve Ozobia, Beale's on-site research director in Mbarara. The child of an American mother and a West African father, Ozobia had grown up on both continents and obtained her Masters in Public Health degree at one of the United States' most prestigious programs. Her self-described "bicultural" identity proved invaluable in her role as the liaison between the American and Ugandan researchers. It also gave her a knack for devising creative responses to logistical problems that the American researchers were unaccustomed to solving.

After considering several options for transporting the blood samples, including using a courier service (too expensive, and possibly unreliable) and a private taxi driver (reliable, but still too expensive), Ozobia decided that the best solution was to hire someone who would deliver the samples by bus—an eight- to ten-hour round trip that would need to be made four to five days a week. Although Beale and other U.S. research staff were skeptical that anyone would agree to such a position, Ozobia correctly assured them that it would not be a problem. (When I returned to Mbarara in 2009, I learned that a local man had been doing the job for the past three years. His Ugandan supervisor told me that he had never requested a vacation, never gotten sick, and never missed a day of work during that time). Ozobia also solved the problem of how to keep the samples cold during the trip. This required they be stored with dry ice, which Ozobia learned was only available from Kenya, and could only be purchased in very large, industrial-sized quantities. She solved this problem by brokering a deal with Mbarara's local Coca-Cola bottling plant, which also used dry ice and agreed to sell the study the small amount it needed to keep the samples cool in transit.

The challenges of shipping the blood to Kampala, and Beale and Ozobia's willingness to go out of their way to overcome them, speak to the way in which scientific legitimacy in "global" research is contingent upon the availability of specific technologies—technologies that might more accurately be described as "local" to the United States, Europe, and other wealthy parts of the world (Feierman 2011). Furthermore, the concentration of laboratory technology in Kampala has created new types of inclusions and exclusions within Uganda. Specifically, the co-location of the IDI and a handful of other top-quality labs in or near Kampala has created a distinct geography of power in Ugandan medical science. Because U.S. researchers such as Karl Da Silva locate their research in Kampala in order to take advantage of the city's superior laboratory infrastructure, Ugandan doctors and aspiring researchers working in more rural, "up-country" areas have considerably fewer opportunities to participate in international projects.

For those up-country physicians who do find ways to become involved in research, the dependence on Kampala labs can relegate them to the role of "blood-senders," making it difficult for them to establish an equitable relationship with their collaborators (Fullwiley 2002). For example, Dr. Gregory Odong, the physician from embattled northern Uganda, complained to me that his collaborators (also Ugandan, but based in Kampala) required that all his blood samples be sent to their lab in the capital, even though he had a CD4 machine at his hospital in the northern city of Gulu. I asked him if he felt like a "blood sender." He responded, "That's what I am describing. We're just a blood sender. And we shall not be quoted into their results if they come out." In other words, he and his local colleagues would not be included as authors—thus denied the professional recognition and social capital that comes with publication, despite the fact that they supplied the raw materials (samples) for research.

Laboratories, in other words, are significant not simply in their ability to translate patient bodies into scientific data but also in their physical locations. The geography of laboratories is the geography of scientific networks. For American scientists working in many parts of Africa, state-of-the-art laboratories are essential tools that allow them to maintain their legitimacy in the increasingly molecularized field of global HIV science even as they shift the focus of their work to "resource-poor" locations. For African researchers struggling to find both scientific funding and recognition, these laboratories offer the possibility of entrée into "resource-rich" international science or—in the case of the geographically disadvantaged—further marginalization.

The Means of Scientific Production

The laboratory and its relation to different forms of power have served as rich topics of scholarship in science and technology studies since the 1970s. Early proponents of "laboratory studies" made the case for anthropologists in the laboratory, arguing that social studies of science should not simply examine the institutional politics of science (as had been the case historically) but also the production of scientific knowledge itself (Latour and

Woolgar 1979; Lynch 1985; Knorr-Cetina 1981). Karin Knorr-Cetina describes laboratories as "fact factories" that enable scientists to isolate and manipulate objects in ways not possible in nature. In observing these fact factories, anthropologists and sociologists could witness the generation of scientific knowledge as a product of contingent "local" practices and constraints rather than the discovery of universal natural truths. Thus, for her, "the power of the laboratory is the power of locales" or, in other words, the power of context to shape knowledge (Knorr Cetina 1995, 157). In Latour and Woolgar's seminal lab ethnography *Laboratory Life*, the power of the lab lies in its ability to transform the disorder of the natural world into legible data suitable for the making of scientific arguments (Latour and Woolgar 1979). In addition, some works have examined relationships of power within the laboratory, such as the division of scientific labor (and social capital) between those recognized as "scientists" versus mere "technicians" (Shapin 1989). Most of this earlier work in laboratory studies, as well as science and technology studies more broadly, has focused on scientific politics and practice in wealthy, industrialized parts of the world.

In the postcolonial science studies literature, laboratories take on new meaning as sites of extraction and exchange. In his historical account of Carlton Gadjusek's studies of kuru disease among the Fore people of New Guinea, Warwick Anderson emphasizes the important role played by the laboratory in transforming embodied organs (in this case, brains) belonging to the Fore into autopsied specimens belonging to Gadjusek. For Gadjusek, Anderson argues, the key to exerting his ownership over brains and other biological samples collected from the Fore was to render these objects "scientific" rather than personal, a feat that was accomplished via the laboratory:

> To make a Fore person's brain into one of Gadjusek's kuru brains, it would be necessary to cut the network, to differentiate native and scientific exchange regimes. The principal site at which this transformation took place was the bush laboratory. . . . In the laboratory the scientist applied his tools to the transformation and de-animation of Fore body fluids and tissues—they came in as persons and left as things. (Anderson 2008, 108)

Many of the other recent works examining postcolonial science have also noted its extractive tendencies, in which plants, animals, and human blood and tissues from the global South supply Northern-funded science with valuable specimens and data (Petryna 2009; Sunder Rajan 2006; Lowe 2006; Reardon 2005; Hayden 2003). In this scenario, Southern scientists must guard against being relegated to the position of mere "senders" of blood, samples, or other raw materials, as Dr. Odong described above. Unfortunately, this is not an uncommon scenario within postcolonial science, where too often "those at the margins are allowed to contribute data, while those in centers provide the theories through which scientific reason will be known" (Lowe 2006, 51).

At the same time, the postcolonial laboratory may offer Southern-hemisphere researchers chances for inclusion and scientific opportunity even as it threatens to marginalize them. For example, in her ethnography of a transnational effort to discover pharmaceutically active plants, Cori Hayden describes the contrasting attitudes of different Mexican chemists toward the project's use of a laboratory technique called the brine shrimp assay. This simple test, used to assess the pharmaceutical potential of raw plant material, was viewed disparagingly by a Mexican government scientist, who saw it as allowing Mexican chemists to perform only "basic tasks" while more complex chemical analyses were reserved for scientists in the United States. At the same time, the Mexican biochemists involved in the project viewed their use of the test with pride as it involved chemical work not being done by their Chilean or Argentinean colleagues, who simply collected and sent dried plant samples to their Northern funders (Hayden 2003, 210). The simultaneous threat and opportunity represented by elite postcolonial laboratories was certainly apparent to me in Uganda, where the careers of aspiring Ugandan scientists could be made or foreclosed based on access to facilities like the IDI and the international funding and mentorship networks circulating through them. These "fact factories" are the means of global health scientific production, and access to them signifies access to the professional benefits of inclusion in international science.

Perhaps not surprisingly, valuable laboratory facilities may become crucibles of postcolonial power struggles, with both donor and host nations resisting their collaborators' assertions of control. This was in fact what happened at the IDI, where Ugandan and North American stakeholders would find themselves in a face-off over the laboratory's long-term ownership. According to Max Edwards, the construction of the new Institute building had been partially motivated by a desire to have a "lasting impact" on Makerere Medical School and hospital. However, once it was built, some of the American members of the Institute's governing body resisted ceding its control to Makerere University, as had been previously agreed. Following a somewhat acrimonious series of negotiations, the U.S. foundation that was the fiscal agent and official owner of the building eventually forced the turnover of the IDI to Makerere. As a result, American researchers who once had very easy access to research opportunities through the Institute found themselves having to lobby for attention, "because," as foundation director Richard Swan put it to me, "now [the Ugandans] can decide not to use them." Not long after, the employment contract of the British woman who had been running the IDI laboratory was not renewed, even though she wished to stay. When Eve Ozobia asked a Ugandan colleague about the incident, she was told the Ugandans at the IDI were simply "sick of the *ba-zungu* [white people/Westerners] and their collaborations."

Questions about ownership, control, and the nature and meaning of collaboration would also arise in Mbarara. Not unlike Max Edwards, Dr. Beale envisioned his work as enriching Mbarara's medical school and HIV clinic. This was an accurate vision, given the medical technologies, jobs, and career development opportunities that the project brought with it, and was shared by many of the medical school's faculty and some of the clinic doctors. Nonetheless, as the project expanded, both the potential benefits and the burdens of having international research in Mbarara also grew, fueling resistance to some of the demands of the research project and igniting tensions over the ownership and obligations of global HIV science. Many of these tensions were fed by the project's unintentional but seemingly unavoidable entanglement in the donor-client politics of development and humanitarian aid that have dominated U.S. involvement in Africa in the postcolonial era. It is the negotiation of these dynamics via Dr. Beale's research at the Wellness Clinic that is the focus of my next chapter.

Chapter 4

RESEARCH AND DEVELOPMENT

The years between 2005 and 2009 were marked by massive changes at the Immune Wellness Clinic in Mbarara, wrought by the simultaneous scaling-up of free HIV treatment programs and the rapid growth of an international research presence. Patient enrollment at the clinic nearly doubled following the arrival of free antiretrovirals via PEPFAR and the Global Fund, and by 2009 there were over 7,000 patients receiving regular care, over 5,000 of whom were on ARVs. In addition, the clinic's staff—not only doctors, but nurses, counselors, and laboratory workers—also grew, as did the space occupied by the clinic. This expansion was funded almost entirely by PEPFAR, the larger and wealthier of the two aid programs. In addition to providing free antiretrovirals for nearly 4,000 patients, PEPFAR money also paid for CD4 and viral load testing, drugs for opportunistic infections, salaries for most of the new clinic staff, computers for record keeping and data collection, and a large two-story building, opened in 2006, that became the clinic's new home.

Beale's research presence in Mbarara expanded in tandem with the clinic, outgrowing its original quarters in the renovated shipping container to occupy several spaces around the medical campus, including a small, three-room office building that the research project built for itself. By 2009, in addition to the flagship HIV treatment study, there were nine smaller studies in Mbarara being overseen by Beale or his colleagues. All told, these internationally-funded studies employed nearly seventy people and enrolled over 500 patients. In the small building housing Eve Ozobia's office, a former conference room had been converted to office space shared by three full-time data staff and one soft-spoken college student, who had been hired part-time to run the study's completed surveys through a data scanner, transmitting the information back to the United States. Beale's project had also taken over another larger office building just up the road. Formerly occupied by the local chapter of The AIDS Support Organization (TASO, which had moved to a new building), it now housed several project administrators, a laboratory coordinator, and a host of research assistants. In addition, Beale's grants had paid for the expansion of a building adjacent to the clinic, where his and other studies shared a collection of small rooms that were used for both blood collection and interviewing. A short distance from the clinic and university campus, the global health program at Beale's university was renting and refurbishing a guest house where its faculty, graduate students, and program donors could stay when visiting the Mbarara research site.

Thus, the simultaneous scaling-up of both PEPFAR and Beale's research endeavors significantly impacted not just patient care but also physical and technological infrastructure, employment opportunities, administration, laboratory procedures, and record keeping at the Wellness Clinic. The treatment programs were humanitarian in nature, in that they provided medical assistance aimed at saving lives in an epidemic that was seen as having reached emergency proportions in Africa. Beale's research program was scientific in intent. But the simultaneity of their growth and the fact that they were both characterized by a large influx of American dollars sometimes made them difficult to distinguish from one another on the ground, blurring perceptions of what constituted scientific versus humanitarian activity. The distinction between aid and science was further confused by the fact that PEPFAR required a significant amount of clinical data collection (for accountability purposes) and that both Beale and some of his Ugandan collaborators envisioned his research projects as helping the clinic by both enhancing patient care and building local infrastructure.

In this chapter, I chronicle the transformation of the Immune Wellness Clinic into a site of global HIV research, paying particular attention to the entanglement of scientific activities with medical humanitarianism and economic development. The awkward relationship between science, aid, and development is, I argue, a defining characteristic of global health research. It is also what makes global health an inherently postcolonial endeavor. Since the waning of the colonial era in the second half of the twentieth century, relations between African nations and "the West" have been increasingly defined by the politics of aid and development, in which North American and European countries serve as "donors" to impoverished, formerly colonized "client" nations (Ferguson 1994).[1] For example, in Uganda, nearly half of the national budget is funded by foreign aid (Mwenda 2005). Currently, Ugandans receive biomedical care through a patchwork of government services, private providers (including pharmacists and injectionists), and local and international nongovernmental organizations and charities (Whyte 1991, 1992; Birungi 1998; Mogensen 2005). The HIV epidemic emerged in the context of this patchwork, giving rise not only to an unprecedented, disease-specific international aid response, but also to transnational scientific inquiry previously unmatched in scope and scale. This was academic science, aimed at producing not only useful interventions to fight the epidemic but also conference presentations, journal publications, and grant renewals from bodies like the National Institutes of Health. But as anthropologists and others have described, the value of transnational medical research in Africa often lies as much in its social benefits as in its scientific findings (Kelly and Geissler 2011; Whyte 2011; Kelly 2011; Lairumbi et al. 2012). In Uganda, this foreign-funded research often provided a level of care unavailable from the public health sector—including some

---

1. "Like 'civilization' in the nineteenth century, 'development' is the name not only for a value, but also for a dominant problematic or interpretive grid through which the impoverished regions of the world are known to us" (Ferguson 1994, xiii). It is worth noting that in recent years China has also emerged as a powerful donor in Africa, to the consternation of U.S. and U.K. authorities (McGreal 2007).

of the earliest access to free antiretroviral drugs on the continent (Whyte et al. 2004). Thus, it is perhaps not surprising that these scientific endeavors would be imagined both as a form of medical humanitarianism and, with the funding of new research and health care institutions, a form of economic development.

Existing anthropological work on postcolonial science highlights how the relationships of exchange that characterize any scientific endeavor—exchange of tissue or botanical samples, of blood, of data, of technology and results—are inevitably shaped by the inequalities of the present as well as "haunted" by those of the colonial past (Lowe 2006, 42). In other words, in a postcolonial context, the power dynamics and hierarchies of "normal science" take on additional meaning and complexity, since they are inevitably infused with the politics of national autonomy, "Western" political and economic hegemony, and (often) race. This chapter builds on this work with the aim of understanding how the rise of global health science—and particularly the U.S. AIDS research community's "turn toward Africa"—is impacting doctors and researchers in Uganda, a country in which AIDS has wrought both intense suffering and an unprecedented rush of international resources and economic opportunities.

In Mbarara, the Ugandan doctors and research staff I encountered were ambivalent about the transformation of their semirural HIV clinic into a site of global health science, and they alternately described international money as "opening Uganda's doors" and "killing our health system." Though contradictory, both are fair assessments of the positive and negative impact of the recent influx of (mostly) American dollars into the Ugandan health care sector. In the first part of this chapter, I describe Dr. Beale's creation and "donation" of an electronic patient database to the clinic, and explore how the overlap of scientific and charitable intentions fed into disagreements over ownership of the database and whose interests it served. In the second part of the chapter, I focus on the perspectives of Mbarara clinicians and aspiring researchers, who alternately expressed both gratitude and resentment over the presence of international science—including my own ethnographic research—and aid. Overall, I argue that the entanglement of research with development makes it especially difficult for U.S. and Ugandan physicians and researchers to forge the kind of equitable scientific collaborations to which they all aspire.

Dr. Atuhaire's Register

Dr. John Atuhaire became interested in medicine at a young age. While in secondary school, he so excelled in biology that his father jokingly began addressing him as "doctor." Later, he would serve as a student health prefect at his boarding school, dispensing medications and transporting students to the hospital during the evenings and weekends when the school nurse was not in. During his last years of high school, Dr. Atuhaire lost his father to AIDS. Nonetheless, his father's nickname for him proved prescient, and upon graduating Atuhaire would win a government scholarship to study medicine at MUST.[2] By this time, his mother was also suffering from the disease. It was the late 1990s, and the discovery of effective antiretroviral therapy had already begun to transform the life expectancies of AIDS patients in wealthy countries. Atuhaire knew this, and despite the astronomical cost of the medications, he hoped that by becoming a doctor he might be able to help his mother. "I had a big desire that I would become a doctor, make some money, and be able to start treating her myself. Be able to buy her antiretroviral drugs and be able to give her the medical assistance that she would have loved to find," he told me in 2004. Tragically, she died just three years after his father's passing, and two years before he finished medical school. "She died before I finished, before I became a doctor," he told me. "So I couldn't do much." Even if Atuhaire had been able to complete his training before his mother died, it is unlikely that he would have been able to afford to buy her antiretroviral medications on the low pay public sector doctors in Uganda earn. Atuhaire was well aware of this, but he still wanted to try.[3]

The loss of both his parents to AIDS further fueled Atuhaire's affinity for medicine, and drew him toward work caring for other patients with AIDS. During his one-year clinical internship Atuhaire began rotating through the Immune Wellness Clinic, which Dr. Salter had founded only a couple of years earlier, where he began treating HIV patients. He got along well with

---

2. In Uganda medicine is offered as an undergraduate degree, similarly to the British system.

3. Atuhaire told me that in 1998 a month's worth of antiretroviral medications cost 500,000 Ugandan shillings, or the equivalent of roughly US$250. This was equal to a full month's salary for a medical officer working in the public sector (Matsiko and Kiwanuka 2003).

Salter, and found he excelled at the work. He found that the loss of his parents made him particularly well suited to being an HIV doctor:

> So I basically I know what an HIV patient goes through. Because I have seen my parents go through it. And I think what I should have done for my parents, I should be able now to give it to others who deserve it. That's one of the things that makes me feel comfortable and like the job which I am doing. Because I don't have my parents now, but I'm doing what I should have done today to other people who are having this same problem.

Upon completing his internship, Dr. Salter encouraged him to come and work at the clinic. Although there was no salaried job available at the time of Atuhaire's graduation, there was word that a position would likely be posted soon, so he agreed to work on a volunteer basis until a paid position opened up. At that time, the clinic operated only on Wednesdays and Fridays. Atuhaire made ends meet by working for pay in private clinics during evenings and on days when he was not volunteering. After three months as a volunteer, he applied and was hired to work in the clinic full time. Simultaneously, the clinic expanded its hours to stay open five days a week.

By this time, it was early 2003, and although free antiretrovirals had not arrived yet, generic HIV drugs from India were increasingly available in Uganda. Those whose families could afford the pills began buying them, and the number of Atuhaire's patients on ARVs steadily increased. In addition, the clinic's overall patient load grew rapidly as the possibility of treatment and the expanded clinic hours drew more people to seek care. As the clinic's first full-time employee, Atuhaire identified the need for a systematic way to keep track of the growing number of patients on antiretrovirals. "When I came to the clinic, there was nobody who was officially assigned to take care of the clinic," he told me. "So there was nobody who was like organizing the clinic data. People would just come in and see patients and write in the file and throw the file somewhere. And that was all."

When the Ministry of Health questioned him about the number of patients receiving antiretroviral therapy at the Wellness Clinic, Atuhaire was frustrated with his inability to answer precisely:

> For instance, somebody would come and say, "How many patients did you have on antiretroviral drugs?" And none of us would answer! Someone would

say, "maybe like a hundred?" I would say, "maybe like fifty?" We had patients on ARVs but nobody would go through the files to dig out the information, store it somewhere, ready it for analysis so that you can easily answer
certain questions of what services we are providing, whom we are providing
care for. . . . I said, how can we be providing care to a cohort of patients which
is increasing every day but we have no information that we can analyze?

As a result, Dr. Atuhaire took it upon himself to start a "small register"—
essentially a handwritten ledger book—in which he recorded basic information about all the clinic's patients on antiretroviral therapy. In his entries
he included a patient's name, medical record number, address, sex, medications, and the date he or she started antiretrovirals. Using the register as a
reference, he could now respond accurately to questions about the clinic's
services. He recounted to me:

So if somebody would come to me and say, "What drugs are you offering?"
then I would quickly go to that register and look through and say, "We have
so many, maybe twenty patients, on Triomune; we have ten patients on [the
antiretroviral] efavirenz; we have a group of maybe twenty patients who
started ARVs two years ago." . . . We were able to know how many patients
we have, know what kind of medications that they're taking, know how
many females, know how many males.

A few months after Dr. Atuhaire began keeping the register, he attended an
HIV-medicine training program at the IDI in Kampala, where he made
Dr. Beale's acquaintance. By this time, Beale was searching for a less urban
location where he could relocate his Kampala-based study of ARV treatment and drug resistance. He began asking questions about patients on antiretroviral treatment at the Wellness Clinic, and Dr. Atuhaire brought out
his register to show him the numbers. Beale was impressed, and immediately recognized the research value of the information. He also saw how the
burden of record keeping could easily get out of hand for Atuhaire as the
clinic's enrollment continued to grow. After making a trip to Mbarara to visit
the clinic and meet Dr. Salter and the other medical faculty, Beale proposed
a research collaboration. He would relocate his study to Mbarara, using
patients at the Immune Wellness Clinic as his study subjects. As a part of the
proposal, he offered to create a computerized patient database and donate

it to the clinic with the intention of simultaneously improving patient care and collecting valuable research data.

Donation

Through Atuhaire and Beale's efforts, the clinic's medical records underwent a transformation from clinical files into scientific data. Through this process, the clinic itself was remade into a site of global health research. For Atuhaire, who, unlike Beale, was a full-time practicing clinician with no previous background in research,[4] this transformation seemed to reframe his reflections on the original clinic register he had created. For example, when we spoke in 2004, after the computerized database was initiated, he described his efforts not in terms of a "register" but as "an automated system of saving the data" using a handwritten "spreadsheet" that he described by referencing the Excel software used for the computerized database:

> I came to the clinic, and I took it upon myself that we should now have an automated system of saving the data. We did not have an electronic database, but I designed kind of like, um, an Excel spreadsheet. And then made photocopies of that Excel spreadsheet. And I started recording all the data that patients had in their files.

This shift from medical records to clinic data was not the only transformation wrought by the introduction of the electronic database. In addition, the database worked to reconfigure the ownership of the information collected within it by making Beale's American research team, as the database's creators, claimants to the clinic's records.

As the database grew, its value as a research tool became increasingly obvious to both the Americans and the Ugandan physician-researchers and university administrators at Mbarara medical school. Not only was the database critical to securing scientific grants to support Beale's ongoing research, but it also served to attract new international research projects to the Wellness Clinic. These projects were highly valued by both the clinic and

---

4. Beale was also a clinician, but by this time his clinical practice was very small, and he spent the majority of his time working on research projects.

the university administration because of the resources they brought. These resources included both clinically useful technological infrastructure like machines to measure CD4 counts and viral loads, as well as other benefits such as new well-paid jobs, scientific opportunities for local researchers, prestigious affiliation with well-known foreign research universities, and eventually new clinic buildings and facilities.

Given the benefits and material resources that the U.S.-funded research project brought to the cash-strapped clinic, it is not surprising that Beale's group envisioned their research in both scientific *and* charitable terms. In the words of Eve Ozobia, "We had a research agenda and we had a philanthropic agenda." The electronic database was born out of the research agenda; it was crucial to making the Wellness Clinic a feasible American research site that could both garner grant support from funding organizations like the NIH and produce data suited for publication in top scholarly journals. But the group also had a genuine desire to help the clinic, and they met this philanthropic agenda by giving the database to the clinic as a "donation," one that they perceived would benefit patient care.

When we discussed the database in retrospect in 2009, Ozobia described its early development as "very informal." It was initially drafted by one of Beale's American medical students and developed on a shoestring budget because at the time Beale did not yet have funding to support the project. The student traveled to Mbarara for three weeks and created a simple patient database on his personal laptop, which he then donated (laptop included) to the Wellness Clinic. As Ozobia described it to me, "It was a very casual conversation. 'Oh,' you know, 'we can do this.' 'By the way, we can leave our laptop.' 'By the way, we have a medical student who can do this for three weeks.' 'By the way, we have data management support that can come and help.'"[5] Over time, clinic enrollment grew, and the database became increasingly formalized and detailed. Data management staff from Beale's team in San Francisco traveled back and forth between California and Uganda, working closely with Andrew Byaruhanga, Beale's data manager in Mbarara, to upgrade the system. The arrival of free antiretrovirals in late 2004 caused the number of patients enrolled at the clinic to skyrocket. In

---

5. Marissa Mika (2009) describes a similar informality in her analysis of collaborations between American researchers and the Uganda Cancer Institute in the early 1970s.

Ozobia's words, "Once PEPFAR funds became available and treatment became available, the clinic went from being a 1,000-person clinic to several thousand, overnight." This growth in numbers increased the research value of both the clinic and its database, and Dr. Beale's success began to pique the interest of other international researchers interested in working in Mbarara. The database became an indispensable research tool and the keystone of several successful grant applications.

As Beale's research project director, Ozobia occupied a unique position. She lived in Mbarara and served as the principal interlocutor between Beale and his Ugandan collaborators at the clinic and university. Her personal and family roots in both the United States and Africa proved to be an asset in this role as liaison. But she told me that her identity as both "African" and "American" was also stressful at times when tensions arose between the Americans and Ugandans, as they eventually did over the clinic database. Trouble began to brew in 2005 when two teams of foreign researchers, one American and one Swiss, approached the Immune Wellness Clinic about collaborating. By this time, the clinic and the Department of Internal Medicine were headed by a young Ugandan physician named Iris Akiki. Beale became concerned when the outside researchers approached Akiki but not himself about use of the clinic data. Given that the cost of the database and its upkeep (which had grown considerably with the size of the clinic) were largely paid for by Beale's grant money, his feelings of ownership were not unreasonable. In fact, they were completely normal—even expected— within the parameters of U.S. science, where it is taken for granted that research funding and data ownership go together. However, as Ozobia would remind him, the database had been initiated as a "donation" to the clinic, and, as such, the clinic owned it.

Yet, because of the informal nature in which the database had been initiated, there was no official paperwork documenting its ownership status. In addition, it seems likely that Beale and Akiki had become entangled in the social and affective expectations of reciprocity that often come with gifts, even those framed as development projects or humanitarian donations (Hodžić 2006; Bornstein 2010). In other words, Beale may have unconsciously expected that Akiki would reciprocate his gift of the database by gifting him control over its data in return. Akiki, for her part, had already given Beale something in granting him research access to the clinic's valuable patient cohort, and likely resented his moves to assert scientific ownership over a clinic she directed—especially since she, too, had research aspirations of her own.

In Ozobia's view, the informal way in which the database was first proposed and developed reflected the unequal nature of the partnership between Beale and his Mbarara colleagues. Despite his good intentions, she argued, Beale's desire to "donate" to the Wellness Clinic was problematic in that it positioned his Ugandan collaborators as recipients of charity. Reflecting on the conflict to me, she asserted in what she called her "African voice:" "If you're giving me a handout, you don't see me as an equal." (Or perhaps, I thought, as a fellow scientist.) Had the collaboration been between Beale and an American colleague, she felt that rights to the database would have been explicitly negotiated from the start—something she did not hesitate to say to Beale directly. As a result, the parties involved had to retroactively work out a data-sharing agreement that would both respect the Ugandan clinic's ownership of its patient information and Beale's considerable financial and scientific investment in it. This agreement was eventually achieved, but the conflict engendered lingering feelings of wariness among the collaborators.

Compensation

The conflict over the database was not limited to questions of ownership. In creating the database, the American researchers fundamentally changed the way that clinicians in the HIV clinic recorded patient visits. This was not simply a one-time change, but one that took several iterations as the database structure was refined and its software was updated. For Beale's team—including Andrew Byaruhanga, who as data manager oversaw the process on a daily basis—the transformation from what they perceived as haphazard handwritten clinical notes to orderly, standardized data collection was a source of pride. They developed a visually striking PowerPoint presentation detailing the shift from records written freehand on unlined paper to a computer-generated, research-quality "clinical encounter form," and this became an integral part of professional presentations given by Beale, Byaruhanga, and other colleagues about their work in Mbarara. In the presentation, images of patient medical records taken between 2005 (figure 4) and 2008 (figure 5) provided visual evidence for the transformation of clinical notes into research-quality data.

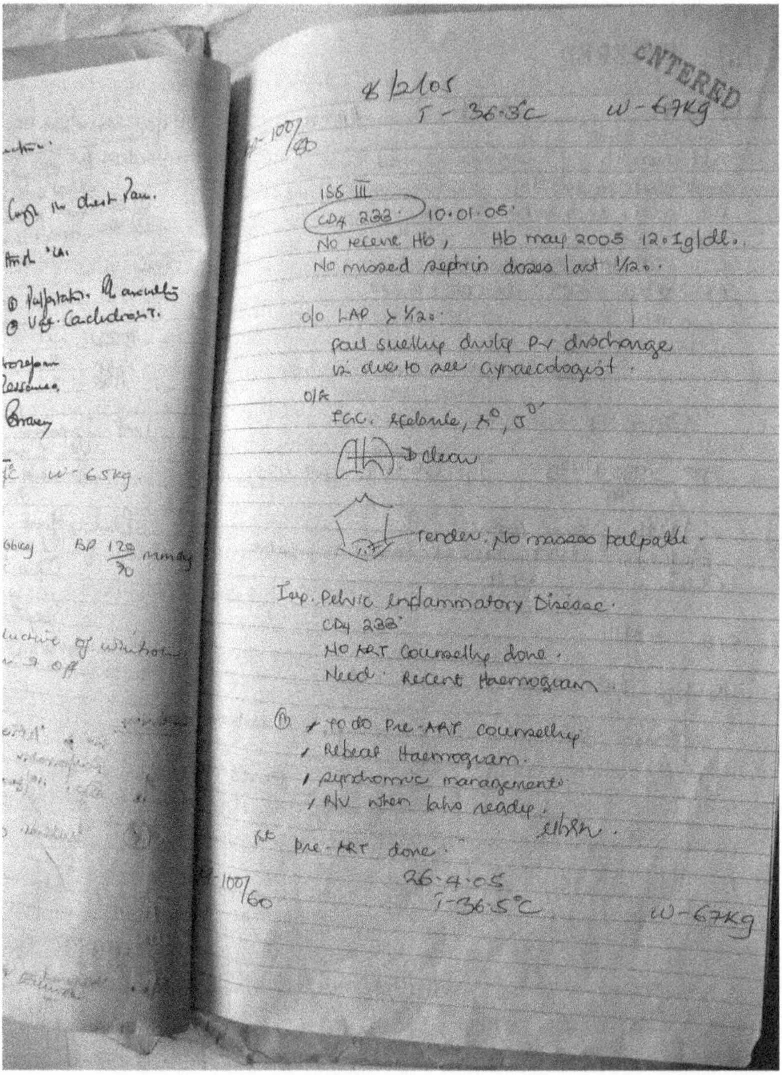

Figure 4: A page from the clinic's 2005 register. (Photo by Michael Kanyesigye.)

In the minds of the researchers, the standardization of medical record keeping necessitated by the database had obvious clinical benefits as well, providing clinicians with an organized, reliable, and current source of information on the patients under their care. This was, after all, why Dr. Atuhaire had begun keeping a register to begin with. In addition, it was through this framing of the database that researchers were able to see their work not only as science, but as a philanthropic venture that aided patient care in an under-resourced setting.

The views of many of the clinicians working within the Wellness Clinic were quite different. Their perspectives speak both to concerns about what turning patients into "data points" does to the work of caregiving (Adams 2010b), and to the social relations of postcolonial scientific collaboration. Although Atuhaire was the clinic's only full-time clinician when the database project began in 2003, a few years later this was no longer the case. The explosion of clinic enrollment due to the arrival of free treatment programs had necessitated the hiring of several other full-time medical officers. In addition, medical faculty at the university rotated through the clinic on a monthly basis. Accustomed to simply recording their visit notes on a blank sheet of paper, some doctors found the increasingly detailed "encounter forms" designed by Beale's data team a time-consuming annoyance.[6] By requiring them to complete highly structured standardized forms rather than write descriptive clinical notes, some doctors in Mbarara felt that the research project was asking them to do research work without compensating them for it. The explanation offered by the American researchers—that the project was in fact "helping them" provide care—did not sit well. Despite the researchers' insistence on the clinical utility of the database, this was not how many of the clinicians initially viewed or experienced the project, which had been implemented with little input from them.

The main exception to this, of course, was Dr. Atuhaire, who served as the American researchers' clinical consultant from the beginning and was also Beale's local applicant to MUST's Institutional Review Board—a

---

6. Susan Reynolds Whyte argues that paper is an important mediator of relationships in Ugandan health care settings, and its use and exchange often enact relations of power (2011). Whyte focuses on the power distinction between care providers ("those who write") and care recipients ("those who are written"), but her observation might also apply here to the relationship between "those who write" (clinicians) and those who "code" (researchers).

Patient ID:	ART Number:

Surname:	Other names:

Treat category	☐ N/A ☐ Orphan Care taker ☐ Health worker ☐ Poor woman ☐ Pregnant ☐ Widow ☐ Spouse of poor woman ☐ JCRC transfer ☐ Other

Address/Phone Change? ☐ No   ☐ Yes *If yes specify new address below*

District:	Sub County/Division:	Parish/Ward:

Village/LC1:	Phone number:	Landlord Name:

Family planning (mark all that apply)	☐ N/A (not sexually active) ☐ none ☐ condoms ☐ oral contraceptive pill ☐ injectible hormones (Depo-provera, etc.) ☐ sterilization/hysterectomy ☐ diaphragm/cervical cap ☐ IUD ☐ natural family / rhythm ☐ other:

Discordance	Any sexual partners in the last 4 weeks known to be HIV-negative? ☐ no ☐ yes

Health education **today?** (mark all that apply)	☐ none ☐ Prevention ☐ Family planning ☐ pMTCT ☐ Discordance ☐ Safe water ☐ ABC ☐ Positive living ☐ Disclosure ☐ VCT ☐ Other

Women only:	**Pregnant now?** ☐ yes ☐ no ☐ unknown If yes: **No months:**_____ **Are you in PMTCT?** ☐ yes ☐ no ☐ unknown If yes: **Which ARVs?** ☐ AZT ☐ NVP ☐ full therapy ☐ unkno **Delivered since last visit?** ☐ no ☐ yes →Date: / / **Has your Infant received NVP or AZT?** ☐ yes ☐ no **Feeding method:** ☐ breast ☐ formula ☐ both

Vital signs:	weight[kg]:	BP: /	temp[°C]:	pulse:	resp rate:

Nurse's name :	Signature:

CURRENT MEDICATIONS (defined as taken during last 7 days)

ARV	☐ Not on ARV's
	If patient was on ARV's since last visit but stopped, why?
	Failure: ☐ clinical failure ☐ immunologic failure ☐ virologic failure
	Toxicity: ☐ anemia/neutropenia ☐ nausea/vomiting ☐ peripheral neuropathy ☐ dizziness ☐ sleep disturbance ☐ lipodystrophy ☐ diarrhoea ☐ rash ☐ liver t
	Misc: ☐ gave away meds ☐ no money ☐ no transport ☐ felt meds no help ☐ felt well enough to s ☐ poor adherence ☐ pregnancy ☐ stockout ☐ new TB tx ☐ finished pMTCT ☐ Other, specify:
	☐ On ARV's (specify):
	☐ AZT (zidovudine) ☐ CBV (AZT/3TC) ☐ NVP (nevirapine) ☐ Atripla (TDF/FTC/EFV) ☐ 3TC (lamivudine) ☐ ABC (abacavir) ☐ EFV (efavirenz) ☐ Other: ☐ D4T 30 (stauvudine) ☐ TDF (tenofovir) ☐ Kaletra (lopinivir/ritonivir or Aluvia) ☐ DDI (didanosine) ☐ Truvada (TDF/FTC) ☐ Triomune 30 (NVP/D4T/3TC)

ARV adherence (last month): ☐ Good(>95%)   ☐ Fair(85-94%)   ☐ Poor(<85%)   **Doses missed:**   **Reason:**

OI Medications		Adherence (non-adherent defined as missed > 5 days in previous 30)	
PCP	☐ none ☐ septrin proph ☐ dapsone proph ☐ septrin tx	☐ adherent ☐ non-adherent	**Reason:**
TB	☐ none ☐ SRHZE ☐ RHZE ☐ EH ☐ RHE ☐ R H ☐ INH	☐ adherent ☐ non-adherent	**Reason:**
CCM	☐ none ☐ diflucan proph ☐ diflucan tx	☐ adherent ☐ non-adherent	**Reason:**

CURRENT SYMPTOMS

Clinical presentation: ☐ no complaints   ☐ complaints
Presenting complaints: *(circle chief complaint, tick other symptoms)*

General	☐ red eyes	☐ vomiting	**LNMP:** ___/___/___	☐ confusion
☐ fever	☐ eye itching	☐ abdominal pain	**Musculoskeletal**	☐ forgetfulness
☐ weight loss	☐ visual difficulties	☐ diarrhea	☐ backache	**Psychiatric**
☐ weight gain	☐ nasal congestion	☐ constipation	☐ joint pains	☐ depression
☐ chills/rigors	☐ running nose	☐ yellow eyes	☐ joint swelling	☐ anxiety
☐ fatigue	☐ nose bleeding	☐ poor appetite	☐ leg swelling	☐ mania
☐ night sweats	**Cardiopulmonary**	**Genitourinary**	☐ muscle pain	☐ hearing voices
HEENT	☐ cough-dry	☐ vaginal discharge	**Nervous system**	☐ other hallucinations
☐ dysphagia	☐ cough-productive	☐ urethral discharge	☐ headache	**Dermatologic**
☐ odynophagia	☐ haemoptysis	☐ genital itching	☐ focal weakness	☐ Skin Lesion / Rash
☐ oral sores	☐ chest pain	☐ dysuria	☐ seizures	Distribution O localized
☐ sore throat	☐ SOB	☐ hematuria	☐ neck stiffness	O general
☐ hearing prob	**Gastrointestinal**	☐ genital warts	☐ numbness	Symptoms O itchy
☐ earache	☐ nausea	☐ genital ulcer(s)	☐ hand/feet pains	O painful

Other symptoms:

ARV **side effects:**	☐ N/A (not on ARVs) ☐ none ☐ nightmares ☐ lipodystrophy ☐ peripheral neuropathy ☐ rash ☐ fatigue ☐ nausea ☐ vomiting ☐ diarrhea ☐ jaundice ☐ dizziness ☐ depression ☐ abdominal pain ☐ Other:

PHYSICAL EXAMINATION

Functional status: ☐ working   ☐ ambulatory   ☐ bed ridden   **Karnofsky:**   %
General exam: ☐ well   ☐ chronically sick appearing   ☐ acutely sick appearing

Oropharynx:	☐ normal	☐ abnormal	**Chest:**	☐ normal	☐ abnormal
Eyes:	☐ normal	☐ abnormal	**Heart:**	☐ normal	☐ abnormal
Lymph nodes:	☐ normal	☐ abnormal	**Abdomen:**	☐ normal	☐ abnormal
Ears:	☐ normal	☐ abnormal	**Urogenital/pevic:**	☐ normal	☐ abnormal
Neck:	☐ normal	☐ abnormal	**Extremities:**	☐ normal	☐ abnormal
Skin:	☐ normal	☐ abnormal	**Psychiatric:**	☐ normal	☐ abnormal
Comments on abnormalities:					

Figure 5: The 2008 patient "encounter form."

ASSESSMENT

Active HIV related diagnoses: (tick all current conditions and highest current stage)

☐ WHO STAGE 1		☐ WHO STAGE 4	
☐	Asymptomatic	☐	HIV wasting Syndrome
☐	Generalized lymphadenopathy	☐	Extrapulmonary TB (includes treatment phase)
☐ WHO STAGE 2		☐	Oral or genital ulcers (HSV) > 1 month duration
☐	Unexplained weight loss of < 10%	☐	CMV retinitis or CMV in other organ system
☐	Recurrent URI (sinusitis, otitis, pharyngitis,etc)	☐	PCP pneumonia
☐	Herpes zoster	☐	Esophageal candidiasis
☐	Angular chelitis	☐	Kaposi's sarcoma (includes treatment phase)
☐	Recurrent oral ulceration	☐	CNS toxoplasmosis
☐	Papular pruritic eruptions	☐	Cryptococcal meningitis/disseminated (inc treatment)
☐	Seborrheic dermatitis	☐	Invasive cervical cancer
☐	Fungal nail infection	☐	Atypical leishmaniasis
☐ WHO STAGE 3		☐	Lymphoma (includes treatment phase)
☐	Unexplained weight loss of > 10%	☐	Recent septicemia
☐	Unexplained chronic diarrhea > 1 month	☐	Recurrent bacterial pneumonia
☐	Unexplained chronic fever > 1 month	☐	HIV encephalopathy
☐	Pulmonary tuberculosis (includes treatment phas	☐	Progressive multifocal leukoencephalopathy
☐	Persistent oral candidiasis	☐	Disseminated non-tuberculous mycobacteria
☐	Necrotizing stomatitis or gingivitis	☐	Cryptosporidiosis or isosporiasis
☐	Hb < 8 g/dl, or ANC< 500 or platelets < 50	☐	Disseminated mycosis
☐	Oral hairy leukoplakia	☐	Symptomatic HIV-nephropathy
☐	Severe bacterial infection (pneumonia, etc)	☐	Symptomatic HIV-associated cardiomyopathy

Other Active Diagnoses for Current Problem List

		4
		5
		6

TB Status: ☐ no signs ☐ suspected ☐ diagnosed ☐ on treatment ☐ completed treatment
If diagnosed/on treatment specify ☐new onset ☐ recurrent/relapse ☐ defaulter ☐ tx failure

PLAN

ARV Plan **Reason** (tick all applicable)

☐ **Continue current**

☐ **No ARV's** — ☐ no indication Indicated, but ☐ defer until TB treatment ☐ patient refusal ☐ on hold for toxicity wash-ou ☐ adherence concerns ☐ stock out ☐ no available active drugs ☐ supporter pending ☐ counselling ongoing

☐ **Start initial regimen**
☐ **Re-start** → ☐Clinical ☐ CD4(_____) ☐ TLC(_____) ☐ pMTCT ☐ PEP
☐ **Book** ☐ Other:

☐ **Switch** — **Failure:** ☐ clinical failure ☐ immunologic failure ☐ virologic failure
☐ **Stop** → **Toxicity:** ☐ anemia/neutropenia ☐ nausea/vomiting ☐ diarrhoea ☐ liver toxicity ☐ peripheral neuropathy ☐ sleep disturbance ☐ lipodystrophy ☐ dizziness ☐ rash

Misc: ☐ poor adherence ☐ pregnancy ☐ stock out ☐ new TB tx
☐ finished pMTCT ☐ Other, specify:

ARV regimen

☐ AZT (zidovudine)	☐ CBV (AZT/3TC)	☐ NVP (nevirapine)	☐ Atripla (TDF/FTC/EFV)
☐ 3TC (lamivudine)	☐ ABC (abacavir)	☐ EFV (efavirenz)	☐ Other:
☐ D4T 30 (stavudine)	☐ TDF (tenofovir)	☐ Kaletra (lopinivir/ritonivir or Aluvia)	
☐ DDI (didanosine)	☐ Truvada (TDF/FTC)	☐ Triomune 30 (NVP/D4T/3TC)	

Provider ☐ MOH ☐ MJAP ☐ TREAT ☐ FTF ☐ TASO ☐ Other:

Counseling Plan
☐ None ☐ First Pre ART ☐ Second Pre ART ☐ Adherence/ongoing ☐ Psychosocial ☐ Other

OI Plan

PCP	☐ none	☐ septrin proph	☐ dapsone proph	☐ septrin tx	☐ other:	☐ stop (Why?: O improvement O toxicity)		
TB	☐ none	☐ SRHZE	☐ RHZE	☐ EH	☐ RHE	☐ RH	☐ INH	☐ other:	☐ stop
CM	☐ none	☐ diflucan proph	☐ diflucan tx	☐ other:	☐ stop (Why?: O improvement O toxicity)			

Other Medications:

1.	2.
3.	4.
5.	6.

Tests ordered: ☐None ☐ CD4 ☐ CBC ☐ Viral load ☐ creatinine ☐ ALT/AST/ALP ☐ CXR ☐ sputum AFB ☐ urine HCG ☐ urinalysis ☐ RPR/VDRL ☐ stool ☐ lipid profile ☐ Others:

Transferred out: ☐ no ☐ yes, to:
Referred: ☐ no ☐ yes, to:
Admission: ☐ none ☐ medical ward ☐ TB ☐ OBS/GYN ☐ psychiatry ☐ emergency ☐ surgica

Other Comments:

Next scheduled appointment date: / / **Provider name:**

requirement intended to mandate the inclusion of Mbarara faculty in foreign-funded research projects.[7] Some of the other doctors felt envious of Atuhaire, whose close involvement with the study provided him with some extra income as well as valuable professional development opportunities (including a six-week clinical research training course in the United States, and tuition for the MPH program at Makerere). If they were going to be doing what felt like extra work for the research project, they wanted to be compensated for it too.

Discomfort

My own anthropological research was not exempt from this politics of compensation. I experienced these dynamics firsthand in the summer of 2009, when I returned to Mbarara to observe Beale's research operation and conduct follow-up interviews with doctors. Prior to my visit I had been in touch with Dr. Mary Balenzi, the Wellness Clinic's director, about my project and received her permission to approach the clinic doctors about being interviewed for my research. Shortly before I arrived, she sent me an email alerting me to a possible problem: she had informed the doctors of my plans, she said, and a number of them had objected, arguing that they should be paid for the interviews. In the United States, given available funds, this would not have been a problem, as it is common practice to provide study participants with reimbursement for their time. In Uganda, however, ethical regulations prohibit payment for research participation. In the context of Uganda's widespread poverty, offering research subjects payment for enrolling in medical studies is viewed as potentially coercive and antithetical to the bioethical principles of patient autonomy and voluntary consent (see Loue, Okello, and Kawuma 1996; Loue and Okello 2000). Such compensation was thus not a component of my research proposal (nor my budget). At the same time, I was also aware that it was a rule that was often bent by providing study participants small amounts of food or other staple goods, money for transportation to the study site, or air time for their mobile phones (Geissler 2011).

---

7. Dr. Atuhaire was also my local IRB applicant.

When Dr. Balenzi sat down with me in her office shortly after my arrival in Mbarara in the summer of 2009, she was apologetic about the reaction of her colleagues. The doctors, she said, were "uncomfortable" with being interviewed without compensation, as they felt that they could otherwise use that time for other things, such as seeing private patients—a common way in which public sector doctors (including herself) supplemented their low government salaries. This kind of demand was new: "It is the beginning of people expressing discomfort," she told me. Indeed, when I had interviewed her and other doctors in Mbarara four years earlier, it had not arisen as a concern. It was not my project alone that generated these feelings, she reassured me, and told me of a Ugandan PhD student from Kampala who had recently asked her to bring some surveys back to the Mbarara doctors for his research. The surveys were thick, she said, and the doctors had protested that they should be compensated for the time spent completing them.

Cognizant of Ugandan regulatory prohibitions against paying research participants, but also aware that small tokens of thanks were not uncommon, Balenzi and I embarked on a careful conversation about what might be appropriate. I suggested the possibility of phone cards for air time on the mobile networks, knowing that Beale's earlier research in Kampala had offered this to clinicians as a way of thanking them for referring their patients to his study. She warned me that there was a risk of insulting people by offering too little, especially the senior doctors who were also lecturers in the university. Offering 5, 10, or even 20 thousand shillings' worth of airtime (about US$10) to a senior lecturer could be "embarrassing," she cautioned me. Then, in a moment of frankness about the racial politics of global health research, she added, "Maybe it would be ok if you were a black." But as a white person, she told me, I would have to offer more.

Our conversation concluded with Dr. Balenzi offering to check with the Dean about whether such compensation was even permissible under the university's rules. We did not hear back from him, but in the end, I was able to interview a number of doctors without offering them any recompense other than my profuse thanks. Those who ignored or put off my requests, I speculate, were those who wanted to be paid or who were otherwise too busy to grant my request. What the situation made clear was that my own anthropological research was shot through with postcolonial power dynamics just as much as Beale's was.

Gratitude

In retrospect, Dr. Balenzi's assertion that "it is the beginning of people expressing discomfort" indicates that my visit in 2009 occurred at a time when the moral economy of international research in Mbarara was shifting. When I had conducted my initial interviews with doctors there in 2005, no one mentioned compensation. Beale's project was still small and relatively new. When seeking interviews with doctors, I found that mentioning Beale's name opened doors for me. This openness was probably due not only to positive feelings about the American research presence, but also favorable feelings about American programs in general. This was in part because the initiation of Beale's research project corresponded nearly exactly with the arrival and expansion of free HIV treatment at the clinic, much of it American-funded. Beginning in late 2004, PEPFAR dollars became increasingly visible at the clinic, not only in the form of ARVs and other drugs, but also computers, laboratory equipment, and new clinical staff paid for by the program. At the same time, Beale's fledgling research study was beginning to enroll more and more of the clinic's patients, and was further augmenting patient care by offering free CD4 counts and viral loads (tests which at the time were often otherwise unavailable).

The Wellness Clinic doctors, who for years had been helplessly watching their patients die for lack of money to buy ARVs, were filled with gratitude for the influx of American resources that suddenly made it possible for them to practice effective HIV medicine. Not only could they now give their patients drugs that would restore them to relative health, but they could also monitor their immunological progress using CD4 tests. For doctors accustomed to working conditions in which even basic antibiotics and simple laboratory tests were often unavailable, it was a chance to finally practice "real" medicine (Wendland 2010). In addition, those doctors who had been hired into newly created PEPFAR-funded positions actually owed their livelihoods to American funding. Thus, on the ground, it was often difficult to tell the difference between American research money and American treatment money. This was driven home for me during a 2005

interview with one of the Wellness Clinic doctors, when she thanked me—
even though she was taking time out of her busy schedule to help me with
my research—thinking that as an American I might have connections to
PEPFAR:

> Maybe what I need to say is to thank God for everybody who is trying to
> help find knowledge about our clinic or about our patients. Not only here
> but maybe Africa as a whole. And trying to help our patients. Our brothers,
> our sisters, our family. I know, because I've seen this work [is] very reward-
> ing. When you see a patient comes in and you know they can't afford the
> drugs, and then they just have to pick them [up for] free from the pharmacy
> at the counter, and then they go home and come back happy, you know.
> Then at least they have some energy to make money and pay school fees for
> their siblings or for their daughters or something like that. I find it very re-
> warding and I think I need to say thank you. *Maybe you might not be directly
> in touch with the people who are concerned, but at least if you are, you're able to
> tell them thank you for the very good work they are doing here. We appreciate it.*
> [emphasis added]

Thus, in 2005, the dominant sentiment attached to the influx of American
funding—both for treatment and research—seemed to be one of gratitude.
Americans were welcomed as generous donors, and Ugandan doctors saw
their clinics and patients as grateful recipients. Indeed, it was this same
moral economy of assistance and gratitude that led Dr. Beale to envision his
research database as a "donation" to the clinic. By 2009, this gratitude was
still present, but it was tempered with a wary self-protectiveness.

In addition to the added employment, buildings, and technological infrastructure that Beale's grants supported, the fiscal power of American research had also become visible in the changing circumstances of its employees. In 2009, Dr. Atuhaire was studying for his master of public health
degree courtesy of a scholarship from Beale's project, and his wife had left
her job as a schoolteacher to become the project manager of Beale's largest
study, a job at which she excelled. The couple, who had been renting a
house near campus in 2005, now owned land and were building a house
there for themselves and their two young daughters. They drove themselves
to work and their elder daughter to school in a Pajero jeep, a step up from
the ubiquitous Toyota Corollas driven by most car-owning Ugandans. Ozobia, who was paid on an American salary scale, had built herself a picturesque

home surrounded by bougainvillea bushes on a hillside overlooking the campus. My friend and colleague Idah Mukyala, who had relocated to Mbarara from Kampala in order to continue working for Beale, was earning enough as the coordinator of several smaller projects to pay a younger cousin's school fees and buy herself a modest secondhand car over the Internet. Given this, it is easy to see why doctors would resent being asked to give their time to research (either by being interviewed, or by filling out "clinical encounter forms") without some form of compensation. Even the chair of the Department of Medicine at the time, a British expatriate doctor, seemed wary of research work that did not pay. Following a lecture by Dr. Norman Musinguzi, a respiratory specialist within the department, he asked the doctor whether he was a principal investigator on the U.S.-funded HIV prevention study he had described in his lecture. The exchange continued as follows:

> Musinguzi: I am a consulting physician.
> Chair: You help them if they have problems?
> Musinguzi: Yes, I help them.
> Chair: [protectively] They are paying you something?
> Musinguzi: Yes, they are paying me something small.
> Chair: Good!

Thus in 2009, as in 2005, on the ground it remained difficult to distinguish between the American dollars brought in by research and those brought in by PEPFAR. But unlike a few years earlier, by 2009 the most palpable sentiment was not one of gratitude but one of guarded self-protection. The longer-term consequences of the influx of American money for AIDS were becoming increasingly visible. These included an internal brain drain of doctors and others out of the public sector to work at better-paid jobs in AIDS research or NGOs, sudden unemployment or cessation of services when a hoped-for foreign grant never materialized, a growing disparity between the state-of-the-art care available at the Wellness Clinic and the lack of even the most basic supplies on the hospital wards, and rising concerns that the world economic crisis and changing global health priorities would temper American largesse and end the era of unlimited ARV treatment slots (which they eventually did; Garrett 2007; McNeil 2010). When I told Idah Mukyala about the doctors' insistence that I pay them for interviews, she told me it was because they could now see that there was a lot of money in research. The doctors wouldn't understand or believe me if I tried to explain that my budget was small, she said, because people think *all* research projects have a lot of money.[8] She told me that it used to be enough to simply offer doctors air time, as she had done when working on Beale's study in Kampala. But now they wanted more—especially, she said, "these PEPFAR doctors," who were accustomed to the higher pay offered by the American treatment program.

Inclusion

This shift from gratitude to self-protection has something important to tell us about the postcolonial power dynamics of global health science. Warwick Anderson describes encountering a "postcolonial melancholy" upon visiting Carleton Gadjusek's former kuru research site in Papua New Guinea. At the height of Gadjusek's activities in the 1960s, foreign scientists and the local Fore people enjoyed a fragile but mutually beneficial moral economy, in which the reciprocal exchange of blood and tissue samples for "cargo" (goods) was embedded within social relations of trust and mutual obligation (Anderson 2008). Years later, things had changed. "When I was there in 2003," Anderson writes, "everybody was talking about compensation:"

> A sort of postcolonial melancholy pervaded conversations, a sense that as individuals and as a people they were unfairly excluded from globalization and its presumed rewards. . . . Kuru research once led development of the region. . . . White men came and went, got *bigpela* prizes and perhaps plenty of money, and left the Fore people with demands unmet and expectations dashed. Now everyone wanted more compensation, especially some of Carleton's former assistants. (Anderson 2008, 215)

In Uganda, too, requests for compensation seemed to stem not only from economic motivations, but from a disappointment with—or a desire to be recognized by—global science. AIDS had placed Uganda at the center of

---

8. My research was supported by travel funds from a postdoctoral fellowship, which paid for little more than my airfare.

global health science, but too often Ugandan scientists remained at the periphery, "excluded from globalization and its presumed rewards," to reiterate Anderson's words. This disenchantment grew more acute as evidence of the economic wealth connected with American research (sometimes elided with American treatment programs) became increasingly visible.

However, what I learned from the doctors who were willing to be interviewed was that money was only part of the picture. Also at stake for these doctors was the issue of *inclusion* in international science, not just in the form of monetary compensation, but as intellectual peers and collaborators. In the sketches that follow, I summarize what some of the Mbarara doctors told me of their feelings about working with foreign researchers, the impact of international research on the clinic, and their own scientific interests and ambitions.

Dr. Douglas Mutungi

"People I think only wanted to be a part of the process."

I interviewed Dr. Douglas Mutungi in one of the minimalist examination rooms in the Wellness Clinic, where he was a full-time clinician supported by PEPFAR. The room contained little other than a wooden desk, which we sat on opposite sides of, and a simple exam table spread with a green sheet marked with the acronym of one of PEPFAR's local partner organizations. Outside, patients gathered on the wooden benches lining each side of the hallway, as they did every morning, waiting to be called for their appointments. When I asked him about the presence of international research at the clinic, he responded with a complaint. The studies were present, he said, but as a clinician he was rarely informed of their plans or activities: "Sometimes you find people telling you they are carrying out a study when you are seated in the clinic and you didn't know what is taking place. They are carrying out a study they never sensitized me about." At times, he would call a patient in to be examined only to find that they had already been summoned for a research appointment, "and I am not even aware of what the project is doing about that person!"

Dr. Mutungi's complaint about international research had to do with inclusion, not money. It was this lack of inclusion that he saw behind his colleagues' insistence on compensation from me and other foreign researchers:

> Like when you had come, Dr. Mary [Balenzi] told me about you and said that people were not cooperating. And I told her that probably the reason is that people come in and ask for information and then come back to tell us what they are finding out, when we don't actually know what has been happening. Maybe that would be the reason why people are not cooperating. It's not you alone [laughs]. There are a number of people who have come here and [the reaction is], "Ah, these people are wasting our time after all. What are they doing? We don't even know." Not that really what people wanted was to be compensated, but people I think only wanted to be part of the process.

Later in the interview, he expressed similar feelings in stronger terms. Most of the HIV clinic doctors were unhappy with the American project, he said. They felt that the research project simply took data out of the charts they wrote up, but didn't keep them informed of the progress or findings of the research on a regular basis. The clinicians didn't feel included, he asserted, and that is why they expressed annoyance to Dr. Balenzi in response to my own requests for interviews.

When I asked about his own research aspirations, Dr. Mutungi described himself to me as "very much interested" in conducting research, and said that he was particularly keen on monitoring the toxicities of antiretroviral drugs, which could include liver and kidney problems, metabolic disorders, nerve damage, and skin conditions. As a clinic doctor, he had no worries about finding adequate numbers of research subjects, telling me, "I won't find difficulties in finding the study subjects since I'm all day dealing with patients." (In this way, aspiring Ugandan researchers may also benefit from the same surfeit of patients that attracts Northern scientists.) However, he thought it was unlikely that he could find adequate laboratory facilities to do the kind of study he wanted to pursue—one that included pharmacokinetic measures of drug levels, and not simply clinical observation of drug side effects. In addition, his appointment as a full-time clinician left him no time to engage in research. Lastly, he would only be able to do research if he were able to obtain funding, which was highly competitive and required finding a senior researcher from abroad who was willing to partner with him, as there were no local sources of scientific funding available.

Dr. Felix Musoke

"It seems you must have contacts."

Dr. Felix Musoke received his bachelor's-level medical degree in Kampala, and in 2009 was in his final year of postgraduate study at the MUST medical school (roughly equivalent to a master's degree in the United States). His clinical duties were primarily on the hospital's inpatient wards, but he also rotated through the various clinics, including the HIV clinic. As a postgraduate student he was expected to conduct independent research. Musoke was interested in blood glucose levels in patients with sepsis, and was studying whether patients' glucose levels upon admission to the hospital had any relation to whether they survived or died. This was a question that had been studied in the "developed world," he told me, "but unfortunately when I did the literature search this study has not been done anywhere in sub-Saharan Africa." It was important, he thought, to see how things might be different in a "tropical set-up" and "in a place where we don't have access to intensive care units or to drugs as often as may be necessary."

Dr. Musoke was paying his own way through graduate school, and had no university scholarships or outside sponsorship to support his educational expenses. Students in his situation were often forced to self-fund their own research projects. Musoke, however, had a stroke of luck. At the time that he was presenting his research proposal, a professor from the University of Virginia was visiting MUST from the United States. The visitor had an interest in sepsis, and asked Musoke to forward him his proposal. The University of Virginia, it turned out, had a partnership with Pfizer Pharmaceuticals to sponsor promising research proposals from Africa. The American professor passed Musoke's proposal on to the Pfizer program, and Pfizer agreed to fund his research. Dr. Musoke saw himself as lucky. "It seems you should have contacts," he told me, "with people who are willing to link you with people who are willing to help you. Because really, if this gentleman had not come in at that particular time, I don't think I would have got sponsorship for my research. If he hadn't come, I was going to put out most aspects of my study because there was no financing. So that's the setback, from an African perspective."

Dr. Julius Katabira

"You need to be attached to someone."

At the time I spoke with Julius Katabira, he had been out of work for six months. The two international studies he had been coordinating had ended. Another one was likely to start soon, and Beale's team was prepping him to manage it, but nothing would be certain until the funding came through. In the meantime, Dr. Katabira was working one day a week at the Wellness Clinic. Although he could have made additional money seeing private patients, he chose not to, telling me that he disliked private practice. Fortunately, his wife had steady work as the laboratory coordinator for Beale's projects, so the couple was able to financially weather his break in employment. And, as he had hoped, the expected funding materialized soon after, and Katabira was hired to oversee a new project testing the use of an electronic pill case to measure patients' adherence to medication.

Dr. Katabira had studied medicine in Mbarara, and then spent a year abroad getting a postgraduate degree in global health in the United Kingdom. After spending some time working in drug regulation and then on a malaria research project, he had begun working as the local coordinator of several projects under Dr. Beale's research umbrella. He was glad to be working in Mbarara rather than in Kampala, and saw Beale as a valuable mentor. "Because I have been working with him, we have been talking and discussing things I'm interested in," he told me. "And I think the idea is that I help him with his work while I learn and also try to do my own things." Katabira was interested in conducting research aimed at improving patient care. "I'm really interested in seeing things work, and really seeing things change for the patients," he told me. Under Beale's mentorship, and with access to the database the research team had built, he wrote an article demonstrating the need for outreach to the significant numbers of patients who waited to seek HIV care until their disease was quite advanced—making ARV treatment less likely to succeed. The article was subsequently published in a top-flight international journal, with Dr. Katabira as first author.

Katabira felt strongly that he would not have gotten the same professional opportunities had he been working in Kampala, where there was an entrenched group of older Ugandan researchers with international connections and few chances for junior investigators to lead studies or author publications. "That's one of the reasons I like it here," he told me. "If I was in Kampala, I wouldn't have written anything or done anything. They will pay you more money, for sure. But you won't get anything apart from the money. If you look at the people in Kampala, in Mulago, they are the same people who were there before we were born! And there is no one really coming up. They are not mentoring other people, bringing up other people."

Mentorship was critical, not only for the grant writing and research skills it offered, but because it was a means of linking into the international scientific networks through which funding and opportunities flowed. To be a successful researcher, Katabira said, "First you need a lot of money, then you need a certain kind of experience and education, and then you need to know people. You need to be attached to someone." For him, Beale had been that person.

Dr. Kizza Mayanja

"You have to dance to the other person's tune."

Dr. Kizza Mayanja was junior faculty within the Mbarara medical school. He had finished his undergraduate medical degree at MUST several years earlier, and then completed a master's degree in infectious disease and clinical biology in the United Kingdom. In his clinical work, he primarily cared for patients with tuberculosis and meningitis, and these diseases were also the focus of his research inquiries. Most of his patients were hospitalized with AIDS on the inpatient wards. Several years earlier, Dr. Mayanja and a colleague at Mbarara medical school realized that the hospital had no protocol for managing patients with cryptococcal meningitis ("crypto")—a common opportunistic infection that comes with AIDS—even though mortality rates from the disease were very high. They teamed up with a visiting lecturer from the United Kingdom and wrote a "small proposal" which they then forwarded to the visitor's colleagues at St. George's Hospital in London. They were then connected with a cryptococcus researcher at the hospital's affiliated medical school, and he helped them secure funding for their initial study.

Since then, Mayanja and his colleague at Mbarara medical school had been testing a variety of different treatments for crypto in an effort to find one that was both effective and affordable given the hospital's minimal budget. The study had been very successful not only at finding alternate treatment options, but also at garnering scientific respect and ongoing support from international funders. Their results had been published in a prestigious international medical journal. Nonetheless, even with this success, Dr. Mayanja felt that his research options were constrained. The crypto study had succeeded in part because it fell within the donors' interest areas: AIDS, TB, and malaria. It was much harder to find support for other areas of research. "I mean, I wanted to look at campylobacter, OK, in this local population here," he told me.[9] "But you can't do that because no one will fund such research. You need specific culture techniques, specific cells, which we don't have here. And no one can give you a fund to even set up a lab that will look at campylobacter, because it isn't a priority."

There were other challenges that came with foreign funding as well. "You have to dance to the other person's tune," he told me. "If they want something done, it has to be done their way, not your way." Also, foreign researchers typically shipped the specimens they collected out of Uganda for analysis. Sometimes these samples would be used for additional research later on, "and we never get to be acknowledged as a part of those researches," he told me. In addition, international research funding was fickle, and studies could sometimes end with little notice due to economic constraints at the funding institution. Nonetheless, Dr. Mayanja's overall sentiment about international research was positive. "The benefits are there," he asserted. "I mean, we've been able to have our infrastructure upgraded, we've gotten very good collaborations, we've written papers. Our patients get drugs—some of these drugs are very expensive! We've actually benefited in that way."

Dr. Norman Musinguzi

"HIV money has somehow killed our health care system."

I first met Dr. Norman Musinguzi in 2005, when he was studying for his postgraduate medical degree at MUST. By 2009 he was faculty in internal

---

9. Campylobacter is a microbe often carried by chickens, and is a major cause of diarrheal disease in Uganda.

medicine, where he taught medical students and saw patients on the hospital wards. In addition, he was "lead clinician" on a U.S.-designed HIV-prevention study located at a rural hospital about an hour away from Mbarara. The project, which was unconnected to Dr. Beale, was funded by the Bill and Melinda Gates Foundation and overseen by the University of Washington. When I asked him what this position involved, he replied that the work consisted primarily of examining patients and filling out "CRFs" or "case report forms":

> We just fill forms, case report forms, which have a lot of information about patients, about social demographics, about examination findings, about history, about everything. There are like ten case report forms every time a patient visits. That's what we fill. We data-fax it to the University of Washington. So we do a lot of data collection, including blood. We fill what we have found in blood, then we fax it also.

The study Dr. Musinguzi describes was actually at the cutting edge of HIV science, examining the possibility that antiretroviral drugs might work to *prevent* HIV infection, rather than only treat it. The findings of other, similar studies were considered landmark upon publication (McNeil 2011a). But for Musinguzi, the work was largely administrative.

In truth, Dr. Musinguzi's primary motivation for commuting forty miles to work on this project was not scientific, but financial. As a doctor who was paid through the Ministry of Health, he simply did not earn enough through clinical and teaching work alone, and research was a way to "make ends meet." Given his choice, Musinguzi would have preferred to work as a full-time clinician, specializing in respiratory disease. But, he told me, "I think the biggest barrier that I've faced is that if I decide to become a [full time] respiratory physician, how will I survive? OK, I'm interested in respiratory—so what? If I am interested, how will I survive from this?" As a Ministry of Health employee, Dr. Musinguzi's salary was low, but he had job security and possibilities for promotion over time. Leaving government employment for full-time research work, he argued, was a poor career option. "If you leave the Ministry of Health," he told me, "you are not promoted. You remain a researcher for two years, and then the project ends, and you are not anyone."

Dr. Musinguzi did have an intellectual interest in research, particularly in research that focused on the respiratory infections he was most interested in clinically. But he was truly a clinician at heart. When I asked him about his own research interests, he told me that while he would be interested in doing research on "TB, pneumonia, cryptococcal diseases in the lung," his "first calling" was really as a clinician. "My first calling, if they give me a lot of money—not a lot, but enough money—is that I sit in a ward and see patients." In other words, in his mind, research work was a good means by which to earn enough money to survive, but he preferred caring for patients over studying them.

Musinguzi spoke pointedly about the impact of the HIV epidemic and foreign aid on Uganda's health care system. "I believe," he told me, "that HIV money and research money has somehow also killed our health system." When I asked him to explain he continued, "If you pay a medical officer[10] more than a professor, what do you expect? It has reduced the level, the involvement of the Ministry of Health." He went on to tell me that even Ministry of Health doctors with the title of "senior consultant"—the highest rung on the Ministry's promotion scale—earned less than medical officers working in research or under PEPFAR. As a junior professor with many steps left to go before earning the title of "senior consultant," this was disheartening for a doctor like Musinguzi, who found himself surrounded by doctors with less training and experience who nonetheless earned higher pay because they worked for foreign research projects or a U.S.-funded treatment program.

Dr. Musinguzi wished that the World Health Organization or African governments would step in and require that international funding be divided up equally among those working in research and in patient care. "They should be getting the same amount of money," he argued. "I don't know how it can be done, but I think where there's a will there's always a way." He continued:

> There can be a way that government can rearrange this, even in Africa as a whole. To make sure these groups which are coming here, funding HIV, funding research, put their money for salaries in one basket so it could be

---

10. A medical officer is a clinician with an undergraduate degree in medicine.

equally distributed. And people in hospitals would be happy, people in health clinics would be happy, people in research would be happy—everyone would be happy. And everyone would now be ready to settle down and do what he does best, and things would be even much better.

Instead, what was happening was what Laurie Garrett and others have described as "internal brain drain"—the abandonment of the public sector health system by doctors and other health care workers in favor of the higher salaries offered by research and foreign NGOs (Garrett 2007). Or, in Dr. Musinguzi's words, "the Ministry of Health people get so demoralized they end up leaving the hospital to go and look for more money."

Dr. Fredrick Muyenje

"We say HIV opened Uganda's doors."

Dr. Frederick Muyenje was one of the most promising young researchers within the Mbarara medical school, and also the one with the most American contacts. After attending medical school in Uganda, he had been accepted into a very selective NIH-funded program that supported his doctoral studies in epidemiology at a prestigious U.S. university. Upon returning to Uganda in 2007, he was hired as faculty within MUST's School of Public Health, a position that freed him from any clinical duties and allowed him to focus exclusively on teaching and research. At the time we spoke, he was studying obstacles to HIV treatment in a nearby rural district, where long distances and high transportation costs often prevented poor patients from making monthly clinic visits to pick up their antiretroviral medications. With his American PhD advisor, he had applied for and received funding to test a mobile pharmacy that would move around the district, allowing patients to "walk, a five- or ten-minute walk, as opposed to a two-hour travel" to the district hospital. The idea had originated in his dissertation research and was now being implemented, with early reports of success. Dr. Muyenje was pleased with the results, but worried about the sustainability of the program once his research funding ended. He also worried about patients' ability to genuinely consent to research, given the extreme shortcomings of their existing health care options. "Viral load testing became available for the first time [in the district] due to my research," he told me. As a result, "I in fact felt guilty consenting patients. Because when we told them we were going to provide a test that was unavailable, that was almost coercion." Nonetheless, he saw that patient care had benefited from the presence of his project.

Dr. Muyenje also had several exciting prospects for new research projects in his future. He was one of two local faculty who had been accepted into a new professional development program that Dr. Beale had initiated through his home university. Called the International Scholars Initiative, the five-year program provided research training, mentorship, and funding support to promising African health professionals. Through the initiative, Muyenje was working closely with Beale on a grant application for a new study of physician retention that would examine how many graduates of Mbarara's medical school had left the country to practice elsewhere.

Dr. Muyenje felt that the training and mentorship he received through both his Ph.D. and the Scholars Initiative were invaluable in developing his research pursuits. It was through these experiences that he had learned the art of grant writing and been introduced to the U.S. "culture of publication," in which scholars' success is often judged by the number of articles they have listed on PubMed. In Uganda, he told me, "We haven't entered into the culture of publication. People do good things and they just have them on their shelves. It's only recently that universities are starting to count how many manuscripts you've written and published." Muyenje particularly valued the fact that he had been afforded the opportunity to work on research proposals from the very beginning. "I don't really like it when somebody comes over [to Uganda] for a collaborating research [project] and he comes with a written proposal," he told me. "I like it if somebody comes with an idea and says, 'OK, I have this idea, how can we work on this?' You see? Then we work together on developing the proposal. Then I take part in that, and take part in everything. But if you come and you say, 'OK, I have this idea and this is my proposal, so are you interested or not—?' Well, you are holding the money!"

Of all the doctors I met in Mbarara, Muyenje was perhaps the best example of a success story from a "development" or "capacity-building" perspective. He had gone to the United States for his Ph.D., but had returned to Uganda to work. His connections with American institutions had allowed him to initiate research projects that were both locally relevant and internationally recognized. The mentorship he received was giving him a growing ability to successfully navigate the world of foreign research funding.

He was on his way to becoming a leader in the field of global health. All of this was made possible because of AIDS, and the way that Uganda's epidemic in particular had drawn foreign resources into his country:

> I think overall we've benefited from the international collaborations, and we are happy that they've happened. You know, we say HIV opened Uganda's doors to a lot of international organizations. If it wasn't because of HIV maybe not many people would have come here. I would maybe not have participated in that training program, an international training program, because it's the AIDS international training program. It's a bad thing that it happened to Uganda but I think it has also exposed the country to certain things that maybe we would never have seen.

Thus, for Dr. Muyenje, not unlike for Dr. Beale, AIDS in Uganda represented both a tragedy and an opportunity.

Collaboration

The obstacles of time, funding, and infrastructure were faced by all the aspiring physician-researchers I spoke with in Mbarara, but they were not insurmountable. As their perspectives show, some doctors were building very promising research careers for themselves on topics that were of great personal interest to them. Others felt forced to do research on AIDS, rather than a topic of their choice, because of donor priorities. Some, like Dr. Mutungi, saw too many barriers to pursuing research and stuck to clinical work, but resented being "out of the loop" when it came to research happening within their own clinic. Still others preferred to work primarily as clinicians, and took supplementary positions in research simply to make ends meet. In other words, the relationships that doctors had to research (and its international networks) were diverse.

In her study of medical education in Malawi, Claire Wendland describes Malawian doctors-in-training as having both a "desire and distaste" for international research work (Wendland 2010, 167). The doctors I spoke with in Uganda were similarly ambivalent: they were grateful for the opportunities and resources that research brought, but also frustrated by the way in which foreign (usually American) control governed their involvement, often requiring them to "dance to the other person's tune," in Kizza Mayanja's phrasing. What their perspectives have in common is a desire for *inclusion*: to be a part of the research discussion, rather than just instruments in the logistical execution of science.

This was a lesson that Beale's team learned through trial and error over the course of the development of the clinic database. For the first several years of the database's existence, the research team faced discontent from many doctors who resented the extra paperwork the project caused them, and were unconvinced by the Americans' insistence that the database was benefitting clinical care. As Eve Ozobia told me, the clinicians' reaction was, "You're asking us to do research, and you're not paying us." It was not until the database software was updated to allow the production of a "patient summary sheet"—a one-page print-out of all a patient's relevant clinical information from previous visits—that doctors began to experience the database as useful to their clinical practice. Dr. Balenzi, the clinic director, explained, "If you have a summary of the latest information about the patient in terms of the CD4, Hb [hemoglobin], clinical stage, drugs given, it helps the clinician not waste too much time looking through the file from the beginning" in order to search for it. Other doctors also spoke favorably of the summary sheet, which by 2009 had become integral to their clinical practice. In retrospect, Ozobia told me that if she had to go through the process over again, she would make sure the patient summary sheet was operational from the start:

> We implemented this database and two years later the summary sheet section started working. And this was the time when the clinicians were saying, "This is a research tool. What are we getting out of this?" They didn't see the relevance. And if I were to do this over again, I would not implement the clinic database until that summary sheet is available. Because the clinicians needed to see the relevance.

In addition to the patient summary sheets, the data team began generating weekly and monthly reports showing how many patients had been seen and how many were scheduled to come. These reports became a key tool in the weekly clinicians' meetings, providing doctors with both a tangible record of the work they had done and a means by which to anticipate and strategize for heavily scheduled clinic days. Moreover, the researchers began including input from more doctors (beyond just Atuhaire) as they continually revised and updated the information the database was designed to collect. One doctor, for example, was interested in learning about rates of circumcision, which had recently been shown to reduce HIV risk in men, so the team added a question about it to the clinical encounter form. All of these steps eventually helped win the clinicians over, giving them a stake in the "donation" they had formerly viewed with resentment.

Similarly, the aspiring researchers I interviewed spoke favorably about international research projects in which they felt they had been genuinely included. For Felix Musoke and Kizza Mayanja, fortuitous connections with international colleagues had allowed them to pursue self-initiated research projects by linking them with funding sources not available locally. Their experiences demonstrate the importance of "contacts," to use Musoke's word, to the success of Ugandan research endeavors. As Julius Katabira told me, it was necessary to "be attached to someone" in order to succeed in the research world. Katabira viewed his own attachment to Beale as a two-way street: he helped Beale run his Mbarara-based studies, and in return Beale mentored him in his own efforts to analyze and publish data collected by the research. For Dr. Muyenje, too, his contacts with both Beale and his U.S. dissertation advisor had been key in opening up research opportunities for him.

Of course, this is nothing new in science. Both "contacts" and mentorship are essential to the success of researchers' careers within the United States as well. In the United States, as in Uganda, junior researchers advance by linking themselves to more established scientists, who have the standing to win grants and get published in top journals. What is different in the cases I describe in this chapter is that the transnational nature of these relationships—and specifically the fact that they are between researchers in a very wealthy country and researchers in a very poor country—embeds them in postcolonial power dynamics steeped in the politics of global health philanthropy. For this reason, actions that might be unremarkable or even expected within the United States—for example, Beale's assumption of ownership over the clinic database he funded, or my interviewees' expectation that they would be compensated for their time—become caught up in a politics of assistance and autonomy that positions Americans as donors and Ugandans as dependent aid recipients or targets of development. This dynamic is further exacerbated by the lack of local funding opportunities in

Uganda, which frequently forces aspiring Ugandan researchers to fund their studies out of their own pockets, and makes linkage to U.S. and European projects an obligatory passage point for Ugandans wishing to conduct ongoing research (Latour 1987). In such a situation, it becomes very challenging to forge relationships that are collaborative. Nonetheless, as I think some of the stories above show, it is certainly not impossible.

In her critique of medical humanitarianism in France, Miriam Ticktin argues that humanitarianism depoliticizes its targets. "The subjects of humanitarianism," she writes, "forever miss the jump to full citizenship" in that they "must remain subjects of benevolence, not of full rights" (Ticktin 2006, 129). Though Ticktin's subject matter (immigration law) differs from mine, her argument is useful here. In envisioning their research in a humanitarian register (as aid), American scientists diminish the possibility of relating to their African counterparts as colleagues. As Mahmood Mamdani has observed, this reduction of collaboration to assistance serves to foster a "consultancy culture" at African universities that discourages the development of independent inquiry and expertise (Mamdani 2011). Furthermore, this humanitarian framing of global health science misrecognizes the value of transnational medical research, which is as much or more about forging mutually beneficial social relationships as it is about providing lifesaving care (Stewart and Sewankambo 2010; Geissler et al. 2008). This is true not only for African research subjects, but for African medical professionals as well. For both patients and professionals, the value of international research lies not just in "mere material benefits or means of survival" but also in "long-term relations and new kinds of belonging" (Geissler 2011, 60). In this register, the social relations of global health science—being "attached to someone," in the words of Dr. Katabira—are about a desire for social collectivity and membership in a scientific community. Similarly, the doctors' desire to be compensated for their time spent being interviewed for my research should be read not as self-interest or greed, but as a moral call for social inclusion in a transnational scientific collective and its attendant economy.

Ticktin's insight into the power dynamic of humanitarianism is remarkably resonant with Eve Ozobia's assertion that "If you're giving me a handout, you don't see me as an equal." For her part, Ozobia was adamant about the need to avoid this dynamic in the future by formalizing any new research agreements with the Immune Wellness Clinic, rather than relying on the informal processes that had led to the initial development of the database (and the subsequent conflicts over it):

> Now what I tell Jason [Beale] is, if we are to ever embark on an institutional collaboration—I don't want to do anything without several meetings, without written documents, without an MOU [memorandum of understanding]. Not just an MOU but a written *plan,* up front, signed by everybody, so that we don't get into the kind of mess that we got into with the clinic database.

It was Ozobia's opinion that this kind of formalization would allow for open negotiation of research terms between all parties, and codify agreements in written documents so as to avert future confusion or disagreements. In her view, the informal way in which the database was initiated would never have taken place in a U.S. context, where all the issues around ownership and control would have been negotiated up front. Significantly, it is just this kind of negotiation that Dr. Muyenje described as critical to meaningful participation and inclusion in research. He resented foreign researchers who appeared with their proposals in hand, looking for local doctors to implement a scientific project they had already designed. What he enjoyed was when researchers approached him as a colleague—someone to bounce an idea off of—and worked with him collaboratively in crafting the shape and focus of the research. He wanted to be included as an architect of global health science, rather than simply an administrative conduit or local stepping stone.

Chapter 5

DOING GLOBAL HEALTH

While in Uganda in 2009, I ended up with an unexpected invitation to have dinner with a group of visiting undergraduate students from a prestigious university in the American Southeast. The students were participating in "The Kampala Project," a one-month volunteer program sponsored by their school and based in the capital city. The theme of the 2009 Kampala Project trip was HIV/AIDS, and, not surprisingly, many of the participating students were on a pre-medical track. One student took a particular interest in me after hearing that I was a medical anthropologist and that my research involved interviewing HIV doctors in Uganda. Over dinner, I listened to this very self-possessed young woman describe her experiences as a volunteer at the IDI's HIV clinic. She excitedly described shadowing the clinic's Ugandan doctors and how, under their supervision, they would sometimes let her conduct initial clinical assessments of patients.

Having done some hospital volunteer work back in the United States, the student was familiar with medical terminology and wielded it with confidence. She recounted how she would examine a patient and recognize herpes zoster (also known as shingles, an opportunistic infection that comes with AIDS) or the skin rash that can be a side effect of the antiretroviral drug nevirapine. She described encountering a patient who seemed dehydrated, prompting her to ask the Ugandan doctor she was shadowing, "Why don't you check his capillary refill?" The doctor (knowingly, it seems) responded, "You try," aware that she would struggle to see results on the patient's dark skin. He also tested her recognition of herpes zoster on a patient, which she had said she thought didn't have the "characteristic redness," by again reminding her that this wouldn't be the case on black skin (the student herself was white). This student was so confident in her abilities and self-possessed in her demeanor that I assumed she was heading into her senior year and likely already at work on applications to medical school. Thus, I was somewhat shocked when she told me that she had just completed her freshman year of college. She was, in other words, a teenager. Towards the end of our conversation, she broke out of her sophisticated medical prose and lapsed into a more adolescent mode of speaking: "What really sucks," she told me, "is that nothing I'm learning will be applicable where I work back home." The urban hospital where she volunteered in the southern U.S. had a very low HIV caseload, she said. Getting to "see 300 HIV patients a day" was something she would never have the chance to do at home.

This student, like increasing numbers of American undergraduates, wanted a global health experience, and the Kampala Project gave her one such opportunity. As such, she is likely not very different from many of the ambitious but well-meaning students who have populated my own classes in medical anthropology. In some ways, she is also not unlike some of the American HIV scientists described in this ethnography. Both were drawn to work in Africa both by a desire to ameliorate bodily suffering and by the unparalleled learning opportunities afforded by ready access to thousands of HIV patients.

Global Health and the New Scramble for Africa

Undergraduate service learning programs and scientific research by top-notch scholars are just two of the diverse kinds of activities that American universities are investing in under the umbrella of "global health." This field, which also includes international clinical training opportunities for U.S. medical students and residents, educational programs for clinicians and researchers in low-income countries, and transnational scientific collaborations between wealthy and poor countries, has seen a dramatic expansion in American academia over the past decade (Merson and Page 2009). As of 2008, nearly half of U.S. medical schools and their affiliated institutions included "initiatives, institutes, centers, or offices" dedicated to "global health" (Crump and Sugarman 2008). Global health courses, majors, and minors have become increasingly "hot" within undergraduate programs (Brown 2008), and in response to student and faculty demand for global health opportunities, universities are both founding new departments and changing the names of existing programs to ally themselves with this emerging field.[1]

A 2009 survey showed that a total of forty-one universities in North America (mostly in the United States) had created "pan-university institutes, centers, and the like" devoted to global health, and that an additional eleven schools had established global health programs within existing departments or divisions (Merson and Page 2009, 3). Furthermore, many schools house student programs and research projects that while clearly of a "global health" nature, are not officially administered by the university's office or department of global health. (For example, the undergraduate program in Kampala described above was overseen by the university's service learning program, not by its Institute of Global Health). Notably, the growth of interest in global health is significant enough that nonacademic entities are seeking to capitalize on it: for example, Seattle's Chamber of Commerce recently launched an organization called the Washington Global Health Alliance in an attempt to harness the city's sizable global health activity—some have called it an "industry"—for local economic development (Paulson 2008; Heim 2010). Similarly, a 2010 conference in Boston touted "New England's Strategic Advantage" in the field of global health, pointing to its high concentration of research institutions and bioscience companies (Powell 2010). Thus, in the United States, "global health"

---

1. For example, the University of Washington established a new Department of Global Health in 2007, and in 2008 the Department of Social Medicine at Harvard changed its name to the Department of Global Health and Social Medicine because, according to its website, it wished to "reflect the growth of interest in global health among students and faculty."

is emerging as a powerful force for mobilizing resources and action both within and outside the academy.

In this final chapter, I focus specifically on the rise of global health within American higher education and academic medicine, with the goal of exploring how the field is producing both new forms of alliance and inequality between academic institutions in the United States and those in the global South, particularly in Africa. In doing so, I draw upon my experiences as a participant-observer at a series of academic global health conferences as well as within Dr. Beale's research program in Uganda. My analysis borrows from Lisa Malkki's concept of "sedentarist metaphysics" in order to emphasize the ways in which global health, as envisioned in the American academy, encourages the mobility of particular bodies while requiring others to remain geographically rooted in place (Malkki 1992). In this scenario, ailing patients in Africa are positioned as offering certain kinds of valuable knowledge opportunities to highly mobile North American students and researchers.

This chapter also represents an effort to interrogate the discourse of "partnership" within academic global health in North America, particularly in relation to institutions in Africa (see also Gerrets 2009). The existence and success of academic global health programs depend upon the ability of U.S. universities to establish ties with clinics, teaching hospitals, and universities in low-income countries willing to serve as hosts for American students, medical residents, and research faculty. Countries in eastern and southern Africa have become some of the most popular locations for U.S. academic global health programs in search of host institutions, as they offer relative political stability as well as an English-speaking elite due to their status as former British colonies. Some partnerships, including one between Johns Hopkins University and Makerere University in Uganda, and another between Indiana University and Moi University in Kenya, are relatively long-standing and predate both PEPFAR and the current wave of global health enthusiasm. Many more, such as the University of California at San Francisco's program at Muhimbili University in Tanzania, the UPenn-Botswana Partnership in Gabarone, Cornell University's relationship with Kilimanjaro Christian Medical College in Moshi, Tanzania, and the Weill Cornell Medical School's partnership with Bugando University College of Health Sciences in Mwanza, Tanzania (recently renamed Weill-Bugando University of Health Sciences), have been established within the last decade.

In the course of my research, more than one American HIV researcher has described the rapidity of this expansion to me with some concern. As U.S. research universities rush to establish partnerships that can give their students and faculty opportunities to work in "resource-poor" African settings, some faculty worry that the juggernaut of global health science is engendering a twenty-first-century academic "scramble for Africa" (Crane 2010b).

Perhaps in response to these postcolonial anxieties, the term "partnership" has emerged as a key word within this new arena or "social world" of global health (Clarke and Star 2003). Host institutions in Africa and elsewhere in the global South are described as "partners," and Northern global health leaders cite "real" or "true" partnership with poor countries as a key factor distinguishing global health from its predecessor fields of international health and tropical medicine, which are seen as having operated in a more top-down, paternalistic mode (Koplan et al. 2009). Nonetheless, in a 2008 article, health scholars from UCSF, the University of Cape Town, and Muhimbili University expressed concern that global health partnerships were being defined primarily by and for Northern institutions. They cautioned, "there is a danger that all this new energy for global health will result in [global health] becoming an activity developed through the lens of rich countries, ostensibly for the benefit of poor countries, but without the key ingredients of a mutually agreed, collaborative endeavor" (MacFarlane, Jacobs, and Kaaya 2008, 384). In its present incarnation, they argued, "global health" risked becoming merely a means by which universities could "brand" themselves in a competitive educational market (ibid., 392). In my own work, time spent among the leadership of this emerging field reveals that "global health" remains an arena shaped by power and inequality, in which the needs and voices of "partner" institutions in the global South are often marginalized and opportunities remain stratified, despite the best intentions of all involved.

"Global Health" as an Ethnographic Object

My concern in this chapter lies primarily with academic global health; in other words, global health activities taking place within universities and medical schools, and which therefore incorporate some kind of commitment

to learning or scientific knowledge production. U.S. universities are investing greater and greater resources into the development of programs related
to global health, and are major competitors for government and foundation
grants aimed at addressing global health needs. The analysis presented here
draws primarily from my experiences as a participant-observer at the meetings of a fledging organization called the Consortium of Universities for
Global Health (CUGH), and is supplemented by relevant information taken
from my fieldwork among U.S. and Ugandan HIV researchers.

The CUGH was founded in 2008 for the purposes of giving North
American universities active in global health a place to share ideas and experiences, and to shape the future of education and research in the field. In
order to become a full member of the organization, a university must house
a multidisciplinary global health program, pay $4,000 in annual dues, and
"have at least one substantive, current, long-term relationship with an international partner university in a low- or middle-income country" (Consortium of Universities for Global Health 2012. (Universities in low-income
countries that have existing partnerships with CUGH universities are able
to join for free.) Initially funded by grants from the Gates and Rockefeller
foundations, by 2011 the Consortium was increasingly supported by membership dues from over fifty North American universities—twice the number of members it had only a year earlier. The number of non–dues paying
"partner members" had also increased in that time, from three to fourteen,
nearly all affiliates of either Johns Hopkins or the University of Washington. The organization's inaugural meeting was held in 2008 in San Francisco, and fifty representatives from twenty universities were invited to
attend. The group's first annual meeting, held one year later in 2009, took
place on the campus of the U.S. National Institutes of Health and was
much larger, with over 250 attendees from more than fifty universities participating. In 2010, the CUGH had its first open meeting (previous meetings
had been by invitation) at the University of Washington in Seattle, and
nearly 900 people attended.

Why study an organization like the CUGH? In a now-classic essay on
the importance of "studying up," Laura Nader urged anthropologists to
turn their ethnographic attention not just to the poor and underprivileged,
but also to institutions of wealth and power. "Anthropologists," she argued,
"have a great deal to contribute to the processes whereby power and respon-

sibility are exercised in the United States" (Nader 1972, 284). The state of anthropology is different now than when Nader first published this piece in 1969, and the subject of power and its exercise is now a major focus of ethnographic studies both in the United States and elsewhere. Nonetheless, her intervention remains relevant, and provides a useful perspective from which to approach "global health" as an ethnographic object.

Although anthropologists have made important contributions to the analysis of postcolonial power relations within global health projects, especially in the field of HIV/AIDS, the ethnographic lens has not usually focused on the field's power brokers. The CUGH brings together some of the most influential individuals and institutions in academic medicine today. Its meetings are populated by prominent and powerful researchers from the most prestigious universities in the United States and Canada, as well as by a select group of elite researchers from low and middle-income countries. This high level of symbolic capital gives the CUGH considerable power over the shape and priorities of global health as a field. Furthermore, this group wields significant influence in both higher education and politics, as was evidenced by the speakers and panelists appearing at the 2009 conference. This meeting included a panel comprised of the presidents of Duke, Emory, Johns Hopkins, the University of Washington, and Boston University, and featured prominent speakers connected to the federal government, including NIH Director Francis Collins, Obama administration Global AIDS Coordinator Eric Goosby, the Office of Management and Budget's Ezekiel Emmanuel (a slot that, on earlier versions of the agenda, was filled by Secretary of State Hillary Clinton), and J. Stephen Morrison from the Center for Strategic and International Studies, a K Street think tank. In addition, the meeting itself was followed by a Congressional briefing. Given its influence, the CUGH is a particularly valuable venue in which to "study up" in global health. In doing so I follow not only Laura Nader's directive, but the urgings of James Pfieffer, Mark Nichter, and the Critical Anthropology of Global Health special interest group, who recently argued that medical anthropologists can make a valuable contribution to redressing inequality by "illuminating the social processes, power relations, development culture, and discourses that drive the global health enterprise" (Pfeiffer and Nichter et al. 2008, 413; see also Janes and Corbett 2009).

The Rise of Global Health

"Global health" is often described as having emerged out of the older fields of tropical medicine and international health, though the question of whether it is truly distinctive is debated, even among those who describe themselves as within the field (Bunyavanich and Walkup 2001). The phrase became increasingly visible in the 1990s, spurred in part by the WHO's efforts to "refashion itself as a coordinator, strategic planner, and leader of 'global health' initiatives" as it attempted reclaim some of the power and visibility it had lost to the World Bank's growing international health programs during the 1980s and 1990s (Brown, Cueto, and Fee 2006, 69). Notably, as a term, "global health" appears most commonly in North America. For example, a 2008 search of the PubMed medical literature database found that 87 percent of articles by authors with affiliations with university global health programs were North American (Macfarlane et al. 2008, 389).

As I described in chapter 1, the field of global health may operate both within a register of protection, in which its primary focus is international health security, and within a register of compassionate aid, in which it concerns itself foremost with the alleviation of suffering and health inequalities. North American universities pursuing global health activities do so primarily within this second register of compassion, pairing it with a scientific mission in which international research and medical education are valorized as humanitarian endeavors ("saving lives"). In the case of HIV/AIDS, these two registers have always coexisted but the salience of each has shifted over time. At the dawn of the treatment era in the mid-1990s, AIDS was emblematic of the emerging infectious diseases worldview (King 2002), demonstrating the globalization of disease, the porousness of borders, and—as described in chapter 1—the threat posed to the American public by potential "super bugs." By contrast, ten years later, AIDS is invoked primarily as a humanitarian concern. Moreover, it seems distinctly rooted in place; its primary symbolic register is not so much global, but African. Within the American academy, the severity of the AIDS epidemic in parts of the African continent is envisioned less as a security threat and more as a scientific and humanitarian opportunity to "do" global health.

The current juggernaut of activity within academic global health has its roots in the U.S. government response to the African AIDS epidemic. PEP-

FAR represents the "largest ever international public health program" (Rottenburg 2009, 424), and, according to its website, the largest expenditure any government has ever made toward a single disease internationally. Because the vast majority of PEPFAR money goes toward funding HIV/AIDS programs in Africa, the program has also ushered in an era of unprecedented involvement in African health by the American state and its collaborating institutions. Significantly, PEPFAR funds travel not only through the State Department and government agencies such as the U.S. Agency for International Development (USAID) and CDC, but also through both public and private U.S. universities. In 2007, three of the top ten PEPFAR grant recipients were American universities engaged in HIV treatment, prevention services, and vaccine research in thirteen different countries, twelve of which were in sub-Saharan Africa.[2] In addition, many other universities work with PEPFAR as "subpartners" to primary grant recipients (AVERT 2008). In this way, the advent of PEPFAR has facilitated the expansion of American academic involvement in public health in Africa by laying some of the institutional groundwork for the scaling-up of global health partnerships between American and African institutions.

Defining Global Health

Since its founding in 2008, the Consortium of Universities for Global Health has emerged as a leading voice in defining and shaping global health as a field, largely due to due to its prominent and well-connected leadership. As numerous science studies scholars have noted, defining the boundaries of what does and does not count as "science" is a powerful act, as it accords legitimacy to certain kinds of knowledge and practice while excluding others (Gieryn 1999). Likewise, as "global health science" rises in scientific prominence and as a funding priority, the ability to define the field—and thus

---

2. In 2007, Harvard University received PEPFAR funds for programs in Botswana, Nigeria, Tanzania, and Vietnam; Columbia University ran PEPFAR-funded projects in Cameroon, Côte d'Ivoire, Ethiopia, Kenya, Mozambique, Nigeria, Rwanda, South Africa, Tanzania, Uganda, and Zambia; and the University of Maryland received PEPFAR funds for a vaccine research program in Nigeria (AVERT 2008).

who and what lie in and outside of it—becomes a consequential exercise in inclusion and exclusion.

One of the priorities of the CUGH's inaugural meeting in 2008 was to produce "a common definition of global health." This definition was later published on behalf of the consortium in a widely cited article in the medical journal *The Lancet* (Koplan et al. 2009). In the published article, the CUGH authors are diligent about distancing global health from the older fields of international health and tropical medicine, which are seen as embodying outdated and paternalistic modes of relating between wealthy and poor nations. As such, they ally their preference for the term "global health" over "international health" to "a shift in philosophy and attitude that emphasizes the mutuality of real partnership, a pooling of expertise and knowledge, and a two-way flow between developed and developing countries" (ibid., 1994). At the 2008 meeting, the lead author of the *Lancet* article made this point somewhat more bluntly, stating, "Global health recognizes that the developed world does not have a monopoly on good ideas." In this way, global health leaders can be seen as positioning the field morally by allying it with an ethic of partnership and equity that the older fields are seen as lacking.

But what if, despite this aspiration to partnership, "global health" is itself an idea of the "resource-rich" world? This possibility is revealed when we compare the *Lancet* article's definition of global health with the CUGH conference discussions that surrounded it. The second morning of the 2008 conference included a panel titled "Perspectives from Our Global Health Partners," which featured the four conference participants who had been invited to represent "partner" institutions in the global South. Of the fifty conference attendees, these were the only scientists not from North American institutions, a fact that did not go unnoticed by some of the Americans. (As one researcher from the Rockefeller Foundation said to me, "If having an international partner is what got us invited to this conference, why weren't we required to bring our partners?") The four international panelists were senior academic researchers from Haiti, Mexico, Bangladesh, and Uganda. The list of their Northern partner institutions read like a check-list of elite American schools—Harvard, Cornell, Johns Hopkins, Columbia, University of Michigan, and UCSF, among others—plus government agencies such as the NIH and USAID. But unlike their American colleagues, who had spent most of the previous day in discussions about how to improve global health education opportunities for their undergraduate and medical students, the international panelists expressed uncertainty and sometimes skepticism regarding the term "global health" itself and what it meant to "do" global health.

For example, Mushtaque Chowdhury, Dean of the School of Public Health at BRAC University in Bangladesh, assured the audience that "what we do in Bangladesh is global health, though we don't call it global health." Mario Rodriguez-Lopez from the National Institute of Public Health in Cuernavaca, Mexico—by his own account, the least well-known of the four panelists—recounted a conversation from the day before with Jeff Koplan, Vice President for Global Health at Emory University and leader of the CUGH's effort to forge a common definition of global health. Koplan had told him, "What you are doing in Mesoamerica is global health!" to which Rodriguez-Lopez responded, "Ah yes, I only just realized it!" Nelson Sewankambo, Professor of Medicine and Principal of the Makerere University College of Health Sciences in Kampala, Uganda, was more confrontational. Sewankambo asserted, "When you see it the way I see it, people are not discussing global health. . . . How do *our* students learn global health? By coming North? By staying home? You need to examine what global health actually means from other countries' perspectives." Jean William Pape, an internationally known AIDS researcher and founder of the Haitian Group for the Study of Kaposi's Sarcoma and Opportunistic Infections (GHESKIO) in Port-au-Prince, echoed these sentiments by arguing in favor of a consortium that was global, rather than North American, in membership, telling the audience, "How can you talk about collaboration when you are thinking one way and you don't even know how the other side is thinking? Yesterday we heard lots of issues relevant to Northern institutions. A *global* consortium is a great idea. You need to include partners early on."

Overall, the partners' comments seemed to reflect that what North American institutions were calling "global health" was simply public health, or "business as usual," in their countries (MacFarlane et al. 2008, 384). If this is so, Sewankambo's question is a provocative one: how *do* students from "host" countries in the South learn global health? One possible answer is that they travel North, requiring Northern universities to reciprocate their global health training programs by hosting students from lower-income countries in Africa, Asia, and Latin America. The dean from BRAC University expressed a desire for such opportunities, but noted that whenever his students tried to travel to the United States they had trouble getting their visas approved (at which point, a Canadian researcher yelled out, "Come to Canada!", eliciting laughter from the audience). Another possibility is that "global health" actually refers strictly to health care delivery and research in poor countries, which puts residents of these countries in the paradoxical position of needing to remain anchored in place in order to participate in "global" health. (This issue also arose during the 2009 CUGH meeting, when a Latin American member of the consortium's Education Committee wondered aloud how Southern institutions might initiate global health partnerships, asking her colleagues, "What do you do, look for an even poorer country to work in?")

This tension over the meaning of global health and who gets to define it was acknowledged by CUGH organizers both during the inaugural conference itself and in the report of the meeting's proceedings that was later published on the consortium's website. In the report—whose author is unnamed—the assertions that "global health is a Northern concept" and that "for the academic institution in the South, everyday public health, medical and nursing education and practices constitute 'global health'" are made on the first page (Consortium of Universities for Global Health 2008). But, significantly, these important points were not included in the much more widely read *Lancet* article that followed the conference, titled "Towards a Common Definition of Global Health," even though this article was coauthored by both Northern and Southern consortium members who attended the meeting, including some of the same researchers who had both made and acknowledged the objections described above. Instead, the *Lancet* article avoids any references to the postcolonial power dynamics of global health and speaks mainly in positive terms of its promise, offering up the following as a suggested definition: "Global health is an area for study, research, and practice that places a priority on improving health and achieving equity in health for all people worldwide" (Koplan et al. 2009, 1995).

Locating Global Health

The question posed by Nelson Sewankambo—"How do *our* students learn global health?"—points to the ways in which "global health" relies upon a version of Lisa Malkki's "sedentarist metaphysics" (Malkki 1992). Malkki defines this way of thinking as the "naturalization of the links between people and place" (ibid., 34). Although she proposed this term in reference to her studies of refugees, her analytic can also be applied here, albeit with some revisions. In her original configuration, issues of nation and indigeneity play a key part in sedentarist metaphysics: certain people belong in certain places—they are "native" or "indigenous" to these lands, and these lands are in turn located within nations that are also naturalized and territorialized as the "homeland." Consequently, displacement or movement away from one's homeland comes to be seen as pathological in that it disrupts or "spoils" the identity of the native, rendering him or her a "rootless" refugee (a narrative she shows refugees challenge with a variety of alternative, hybrid identities). Although the politics of indigeneity and nation do not play out as strongly in the sedentarist metaphysics I attribute to "global health," there are nonetheless significant and largely unspoken assumptions about people (specifically, bodies) and places underlying the field, its structure, and its practices. More precisely, global health relies upon a very strong notion of *bodies in place* in which certain kinds of patient bodies are linked to certain kinds of places, and, by extension, certain kinds of biomedical learning opportunities.

In the United States, many university-based global health programs emphasize the importance of hands-on international experience. At Cornell University, which established an instantly popular undergraduate minor in global health in 2007, students participating in the global health program are required to complete an eight-week internship abroad in a "resource-poor" setting (Cornell University Division of Nutritional Sciences 2012). At UCSF, graduate students in the Global Health Clinical Scholars Program "generally spend a minimum of one month in a resource-scarce country practicing clinical medicine, conducting a research project, or participating in program development" (UCSF Global Health Sciences 2012). And at Duke University's medical school, third-year medical students participating in the Global Health Study Program are linked with research opportunities at the university's various "global health international field sites," while medical residents are offered the chance to provide care in a "resource-constrained setting and conduct research at a partnering global health site" (Duke University School of Medicine 2012; Duke Global Health Institute 2012). All of these programs, as well as others like them, are enabled by the mobility of Northern researchers and students, who are both willing and able to travel across continents to achieve certain kinds of experiences, training, and research opportunities. The value and authenticity of these global health experiences, in turn, is contingent upon the availability of certain kinds of bodies located in certain kinds of places. Southern patients and their ailments are envisioned as biological embodiments of settings alternately described as "resource-poor," "resource-scarce," and "resource-constrained," and working with them represents the chance to "do" global health. Thus, within academic global health in North America, the availability of patient bodies—lots of them—suffering from high levels of illness (especially infectious disease) and low levels of pharmaceutical, surgical, and other forms of treatment is both an inequality to be redressed and an opportunity to be taken advantage of.

Of course, patient bodies are not the only bodies to consider here. The bodies of North American students and faculty are highly mobile, and their ease of global travel contrasts sharply with the difficulties faced by many of their Southern peers, who despite their middle-class status face both financial and political barriers to international travel and learning. This is evident in Mushtaque Chowdury's complaint, cited earlier, about the visa troubles his Bangladeshi medical students experience when attempting to travel to the United States. It also arose in complaints voiced by Americans at the CUGH conference regarding the difficulty of establishing reciprocal exchanges with Southern institutions. For example, at the 2009 meeting, a representative from the University of Minnesota told me that his attempts to host foreign medical residents were thwarted by the university's teaching hospital, which "puts up so many hurdles that it's almost impossible," including forbidding foreign medical residents from seeing patients, even though they are brought over under the auspices of the medical school. This contrasts sharply with the ease with which even low-level undergraduate students from the United States are able to access the bodies of patients in the countries hosting them, as demonstrated in my opening vignette from Kampala (see also Brada 2011b; Wendland 2012).

A Resource in Refugees

The implicit linkage of bodies and places in global health is also visible in debates over what "counts" as a global health experience, and specifically whether or not it is possible to "do" global health in the United States. This was an issue in the planning of Cornell University's undergraduate global health minor several years ago, where it was ultimately decided that the program would require an international internship. Other programs have gone the other way and chosen to include certain kinds of work within the United States under the rubric of global health. For example, students wanting to earn a master of science in global health from UCSF are permitted to conduct their required field experience with a "local underserved population." At the CUGH's 2009 annual meeting, the question of whether domestic work counted as global health was a topic of active discussion. Representatives of programs that recognized North American work as "global health" advocated the utility of the United States' diversity in this regard. One doctor from Oregon Health Sciences University promoted the usefulness of immigrant patients for medical student learning, noting, "We've found a resource in refugees," and advocated, "We need to invest in this population as a part of global health." A colleague from Boston University concurred, saying, "We're so diverse, global health is right outside our door."

Another example of this "refugees as resource" approach can be seen on the website of the University of Minnesota Medical School, which in 2010 promoted its International Medical Education and Research Program by touting the abundance of immigrant and refugee communities and their associated "tropical diseases" in Minnesota:

> Minnesota has become recognized as an epicenter in the field of Immigrant Health due to a major influx of immigrants in the 1980's and 90's from Southeast Asia, Latin America, and Africa. Indeed you don't have to leave Minnesota to see patients with "tropical diseases", such as malaria, strongyloidiasis, or buruli ulcer—even in January! Tuberculosis, which is declining in most states, has not abated in Minnesota, with over 75% of cases occurring among the foreign born. Over 400 immigrants with HIV/AIDS are cared for at clinics within the Twin Cities, which has become a microcosm of this devastating epidemic in their homeland (University of Minnesota Medical School 2010).

In a subsequent paragraph, readers were informed that the medical school had undertaken "major changes" in its curriculum to reflect the changing demographics of the state, including the development of a "Global Health Pathway" for entering medical students wanting to pursue work in international medicine.

While these statements promoting U.S.-based study may at first seem to contradict my assertion that global health depends upon certain kinds of "bodies in place," I would argue that the emphasis on refugees and immigrants suggests otherwise. Instead, within the global health imaginary, such patients are seen as biomedical embodiments of the "resource-poor" geographies from whence they came. In other words, they bring the "global" with them, and can thus be seen as representing an "Other" or "exotic within" the United States.[3] Given this, it will be interesting to see how global health programs evolve and whether or not work with impoverished U.S. populations—especially the U.S.-born—gains wide acceptance as a legitimate global health experience. This question is not merely semantic, as the explosion in global health–related funding puts projects and activities able to position themselves as within global health at a distinct advantage for support. More importantly, it has consequences for the bodily survival of patients who receive services through such programs.

Certainly within the field of HIV/AIDS, public and academic attention to the epidemic abroad (particularly in Africa), seems to currently exceed interest in HIV at home—a striking development, given that HIV in Africa received little attention from the United States during the first decade and a half of the epidemic. Now, in a remarkable shift, the African American community—one of the U.S. groups hardest hit by HIV—has begun comparing its HIV rates to those in Africa in an attempt to garner increased government attention and support. Here I refer to the 2008 report issued by the Los Angeles-based Black AIDS Institute with the noteworthy title, "Left Behind: Black America—A Neglected Priority in the Global AIDS Epidemic." The report includes a full-page silhouette image of the west African nation of Côte D'Ivoire accompanied by the statement, "If Black America was a country, its AIDS epidemic would be nearly the size of the AIDS epidemic in Côte D'Ivoire" (Wilson, Wright and Isbell 2008, 6). On the previous page, the report states, "the number of people living with HIV in Black America exceeds the HIV populations in 7 of the 15 focus countries of the U.S. government's PEPFAR initiative." Whether this advocacy organization succeeds in gaining recognition for African Americans with HIV as a "global health" population remains to be seen. However, it is worth

---

3. I borrow the phrase "exotic within" from Sindhu Revuluri.

noting that, following the publication of this report, the director of Columbia University's International Center for AIDS Care and Treatment Program, which works in thirteen African countries, authored an article in the *New England Journal of Medicine* decrying the "forgotten" epidemic in the United States, particularly among "poor black Americans" (El-Sadr, Mayer, and Hodder 2010).

Postcolonial Partnership

Global health envisions African patients not just as persons in need of treatment, but also as "bodies of knowledge" capable of yielding valuable scientific information. This, in itself, does not make them different from patients participating in medical research in the United States or elsewhere. Research subjects and research scientists everywhere must balance between the clinical imperative to heal and the scientific priority of data production. What makes global health research different is the radical inequality and geographic distance that underpin it, leaving the field haunted by a postcolonial power differential that it continually struggles against. In this context, the discourse of "partnership" between Northern and Southern institutions has emerged as a key strategy for confronting, at least rhetorically, the problem of inequality.

Aspiring academic global health researchers in the North are acutely aware of the dubious ethical conditions under which earlier international research was carried out. In the colonial and post-independence eras, American and European scientists often simply collected the data they wanted and left, with little accountability to Southern host communities, institutions, or researchers. In global health circles, this style of science is referred to as "parachute," "helicopter," or "safari" research, and looked upon disapprovingly. Instead, "partnership" with scientists and institutions in poor countries is advocated as an alternative, more equitable approach to conducting international research. Most often, this call to collaborate is aimed at African universities, which make up the bulk of global health partnership agreements with North American institutions (CSIS 2009).

Partnership between American and African institutions provides U.S. researchers with access to desirable patient populations, as well as African colleagues qualified to shepherd proposals through local IRB approval. At the same time, partnership offers genuine benefits to African host institutions, including investment in infrastructure (such as laboratories, information technology, and buildings), job creation, and funded research opportunities for African investigators such as those in Mbarara, who might otherwise have little access to scientific grants. Many global health partnerships espouse an explicit commitment to "capacity-building" and offer training in research skills to African physicians, with the goal of fostering local expertise and leadership in global health science. Dr. Beale's International Scholars Initiative, which provided advanced research training and mentorship to Dr. Frederick Muyenje and other promising young investigators at MUST, is one example of such a benefit. Thus, "partnership" is not an empty promise, and there are many ways in which these alliances are mutually beneficial. At the same time, however, significant inequalities persist, and the promotion of global health by Northern stakeholders as a "win-win" example of genuine partnership risks obscuring this. As Rene Gerrets notes in his work on public-private partnerships in global health, "the notion of 'partnership' and its emphasis on equality and consensus, stands at odds with the diverse social realities and dynamics among the sites and actors that global health partnerships typically engage" (Gerrets 2010).

Within the context of the CUGH meetings, the term "partnership" played a prominent role, serving as a defining characteristic of the field of global health, a descriptor of the role played by Southern institutions and experts, and a qualifying condition for membership in the consortium. In addition, when meeting attendees described challenges or inequalities they had encountered in their global health work, "partnership" was often proposed as the remedy. For example, one U.S. university president speaking at the 2009 meeting noted the need for "humility" in the face of global health interventions that had been unsuccessful. Citing an instance in which donors had failed to realize that Sudanese recipients of insecticide-treated bed nets would want to wash the nets in order to remove the cooking smoke they collected (thus also removing the insecticide), he asked, "How will we do better in the future? By partnering with the people it impacts." In a different mode, at the same meeting, an NIH scientist described the reluctance of some U.S. institutions to participate in global health research out of fear of losing grant money to foreign collaborators. This anxiety could be assuaged, she said, by funding "partnerships" between domestic and foreign universities. In juxtaposing these two examples, we can see that the same concept of "partnership" is being used to describe very different things: in the first case, a call for community-based public health intervention, and in the second, the creation of a transnational institutional structure for the purposes of administering research funds.

However, despite the frequent invocation of the idea of "partnership" in global health, the field has given little consideration to what partnership actually entails in practice or to the wide variety of relationships that currently exist between Northern and Southern entities. This lack of attention to the meanings and activities taking place in the name of partnership risks obscuring the diversity of arrangements and complex power dynamics at stake. Below, an examination of some of the administrative mechanisms behind global health partnership reveals ongoing tensions between Northern and Southern perspectives, and uncertainty over whether these partnerships benefit or deplete host institutions.

The (Indirect) Costs of Partnership

At the CUGH meetings, the priorities of partnership seemed different for the North American conference organizers and for the small group of Southern invitees. While panelists from Southern institutions tended to prioritize issues of equity and opportunity in their partnerships with North American schools—such as having a voice in research priorities, giving their students overseas learning opportunities, and building capacity at their home institutions—American panelists spent more time focused on the logistics of transnational academic collaboration, and particularly the navigation of complex bureaucracies of both U.S. and host institutions. Potentially controversial topics such as the efficient and legal movement of money, compensation rates for foreign employees, compliance with national tax laws abroad, intellectual property rights, and ethical approval for research were all discussed within the deceptively bland vocabulary of "enabling systems," "harmonization," and the establishment of a "common platform."

The value that Northern institutions placed on administrative streamlining was evident at the CUGH's inaugural meeting in 2008, where the unexpected star of the conference was not a high-profile researcher but a University of Washington administrator who was one of the very few presenters without a graduate degree. The administrator wowed the audience of MDs and PhDs with her description of the administrative prowess of the UW's Global Support Project (GSP), which she had spearheaded in 2007 in order to coordinate and facilitate the university's increasing number of projects abroad by "optimiz[ing] the administrative processes that support global research and education" (University of Washington 2007, 1). She began her presentation to the CUGH with the assertion that "normal is defined differently everywhere," giving the example that what is normal in Seattle might not be considered normal in Ethiopia. She underscored this point by showing the audience a humorous photo depicting a group of people seated at an outdoor table, nonchalantly chatting and sipping beverages as several zebras drank from the swimming pool a few feet away—an apparently "normal" event in Kenya, where the photo was taken.

According to the administrator, the Global Support Program came about in response to the discovery that university scientists were running their global health projects out of personal bank accounts because the University of Washington (UW) did not offer the administrative structures they needed to manage international research. For example, UW did not have a mechanism for transferring more than $50,000 to a foreign country, even though administrative offices were getting requests for amounts in the range of $250,000 from principal investigators running studies overseas. As a result, projects were having serious problems getting cash to their local staff for hiring and operating expenses. The Global Support Project was designed to establish structures that could handle this kind of transnational fiscal administration, as well as issues like in-country subcontracting and human resources, tax compliance, information technology infrastructure, and risk and emergency management. Included in the GSP's services was assistance establishing "shell" nongovernmental organizations (NGOs) in host countries to act as fiscal and legal agents for global health projects, as the university was not permitted to register as a nonprofit abroad. In addition, as part of the Global Support Project, Seattle-based administrators were sent overseas to visit the university's international field sites—what the speaker described as "sending accountants on a road tour of Africa"—in order to give them a sense of "what goes on on the ground." Furthermore, as a state university, the GSP also worked locally to forge "relationships with people in the state capitol and get them on board," even succeeding in getting some state laws changed to facilitate their work.

Overall, the presenter painted a picture of a powerful, well-oiled administrative apparatus staffed by what she termed "fearless provocateurs" and dedicated to facilitating efficient and responsible international work. The motto of the GSP, she said, is "We Help People Who Change the World." Her presentation was very well received, and led to speaking invitations from other North American campuses seeking to replicate the Global Support Project, as well as an invitation to lead the meeting on "Enabling Platforms" at the CUGH again the following year. (At this subsequent meeting King Holmes, the chair of UW's Department of Global Health, would introduce her to the audience as "our savior.")

However, when North American meeting organizers asked representatives from Southern "partner" institutions whether it would be useful to share the GSP administrator's expertise with international staff, the response was more mixed. Jean William Pape, the Haitian researcher, agreed that it would indeed be "very useful." But Ugandan scholar Nelson Sewankambo disagreed, arguing that Northern universities were "undermining local capacity" by setting up separate administrative bodies in NGO form, rather than utilizing existing local administrative structures. The University of Washington NGO in Addis Ababa, Ethiopia, he argued, was undermining capacity at their partner institution, the University of Addis Ababa. Instead of establishing their own NGO to handle the grant money, he said, "They need to help the University of Addis Ababa manage the finances." Tom Quinn, the founding director of the Johns Hopkins Center for Global Health and a long-term collaborator of Sewankambo's, echoed this sentiment. "I agree that's happening a lot," he told the audience. International projects were building outside structures, he said, because local ones are "too difficult."[4]

---

4. While government and university bureaucracies (both foreign and domestic) can certainly pose unwanted challenges and delays to eager researchers, the circumvention of African management and regulatory structures can also work to exclude and marginalize African experts from global health planning and governance. As Elise Carpenter has noted in her study of Botswana's national HIV treatment program (established through a government partnership with Harvard University and Merck Pharmaceuticals), "In most portrayals of Botswana's HIV [program] by international experts or donor organizations, barriers are called bureaucracy, success is called partnership. This effectively negates the contributions of [Botswanan] government bureaucrats" (Carpenter 2010).

This exchange reflects a much larger and ongoing debate in global health over whether Northern funding is helping to improve local health and education systems in Africa and elsewhere, or undermining them by setting up parallel, largely independent structures.[5] While most North American global health endeavors cite "capacity-building" at partner institutions as one of their goals, this is usually envisioned in the form of training opportunities for local researchers and clinicians and infrastructural improvements to buildings, laboratories, and information technology—not in terms of fiscal administration. However, global health projects are undoubtedly straining the fiscal capacities of partner institutions, which were not designed to administer huge scientific grants from the American government. During the 2008 CUGH meeting, one American researcher said to me in an aside that his university's program in Botswana had received "one grant that was bigger than the whole local university budget," which had, not surprisingly given its size, "no idea how to manage it." It's a real problem, he went on, because they "desperately want to be treated like equals" but are not able to handle large NIH grants.

The challenge of handling large sums of grant money is exacerbated by NIH regulations, which cap reimbursements for "indirect costs"—i.e., administrative and infrastructural overhead—at 8 percent for foreign institutions. By contrast, American institutions, which negotiate this rate with the NIH individually, are reimbursed for indirect costs at much higher rates: for example, the website for the Johns Hopkins School of Medicine lists a 62 percent reimbursement rate for federally funded research conducted on campus. In other words, if the medical school were to receive an NIH grant for $100,000, another $62,000 would be added on to this to cover "indirect" overhead costs. A foreign university receiving a grant of the same size

---

5. With its vertical administrative structure and heavy usage of U.S. subcontractors for supply chain management, PEPFAR has been particularly controversial in this regard. At the Immune Wellness Clinic, the PEPFAR-run antiretroviral programs are undoubtedly more reliable and successful than programs run through the Ugandan Ministry of Health, which suffer from interruptions in drug supply, less optimal drug choices, and less availability of CD4 and viral load testing. This has served to increase confidence in foreign-funded projects and fueled existing discontent with the efficiency and reliability of government programs in Uganda. Of course, PEPFAR is also much better funded. The question at stake is whether investing U.S. funds in Ministry of Health systems instead of creating the largely independent PEPFAR program could result in successful government-run treatment programs.

would only be given $8,000 to cover administrative expenses. This 8 percent reimbursement is actually an improvement over NIH regulations in the 1980s, which did not allow any indirect cost reimbursements for foreign institutions—a product of negative Reagan-era sentiments toward foreign aid. The rule changed in the 1990s, when fears of "emerging diseases" made the climate for international health funding more favorable. Officials at the National Institutes of Allergy and Infectious Disease successfully lobbied for an increase to 8 percent, the same amount that the NIH offers recipients of its training grants, but found that any amount greater than this was politically untenable (John McGowan and Gray Handley, personal communication). The consequence is that universities in low-income countries in Africa and elsewhere are being asked to manage large scientific grants from the U.S. government, but are offered insufficient reimbursement for the administrative costs of doing so—a recipe that sets them up for failure. I witnessed this in my own research, where the NGO established to serve as the Ugandan fiscal agent for Dr. Beale's research suffered a financial meltdown as U.S. interest in conducting research at the site grew and the number of projects it was expected to administer ballooned beyond its capacity.

This problem did not go unrecognized at the CUGH meeting, where one American scientist noted that the low reimbursement rate was simply not enough for foreign universities to build the infrastructure needed to support international partnership. An 8 percent reimbursement rate, he said, was simply "not very partner-like." This challenges the public promotion of global health partnerships as inherently mutually beneficial, and raises an important question: does the language of partnership serve as an obfuscation, turning our attention away from the inequalities that are produced when North American global health programs seek to streamline access to the bodies of Southern patients?

Valuable Inequalities

Given the ongoing context of global socioeconomic inequality, how might these emerging disparities within global health programs and practice be ameliorated? Clearly, efforts to define the meaning, scope, and mission of global health need to be more inclusive of perspectives from low-income nations—otherwise, claims of partnership are likely to remain strictly aspirational rather than actual. To do this, scholars from poor and middle-income countries need to be included in larger numbers and at higher levels in organizations like the CUGH, lest such groups become de facto clubs of North American academic power brokers. At the CUGH meetings, there was some awareness of this problem among North American participants. In a discussion toward the closing of the 2009 meeting concerning the membership status of Southern "partner" institutions, one CUGH board member noted that "there is lots of discussion about how low- and middle-income partners should participate, but there are no representatives *from* a partner institution in the room." The 2010 meeting in Seattle, which had both greater overall attendance and more international participants, showed some improvement on this front, perhaps due to its more open attendance policy.

However, the challenges to equity within global health go beyond issues of definition and representation. In addition to making global health more inclusive, North American universities must come to terms with the fact that the very poverty and inequality they aspire to remedy is also what makes their global health programs both possible and popular. In other words, in the world of academic global health, inequality is a valuable opportunity. In her work on the globalization of clinical trials research, Adriana Petryna has shown how the for-profit research sector is exploiting this opportunity by seeking out lower-income countries as locations for pharmaceutical testing. Countries like Brazil and Poland, she writes, allow trials to be conducted more cheaply and efficiently than is possible in the United States, due to their large numbers of untreated patients and variable ethical requirements (Petryna 2009). The global health activities I have described here bear both important similarities and differences to the private-sector research described by Petryna. A key difference is that academic global health research is largely federally funded and aimed at producing scientific and public health knowledge useful and applicable primarily in the South, not the North, where different standards of care preclude the testing of many interventions designed for impoverished settings (Crane 2010, Wendland 2008). In addition, unlike the international science studied by Petryna, academic global health is not limited to research, as it also encompasses clinical training activities for health professionals and students from both sponsor and host nations.

But there are other ways in which global health enthusiasts in the academy resemble their colleagues in the private sector, most notably in the way in which they benefit from the opportunities afforded by global inequalities. Petryna describes how lack of oversight of international clinical trials, combined with health system inadequacies in lower- and middle-income countries, permit a kind of "experimentality" in which "experiments draw from public resources and are coined as social goods" (Petryna 2009, 30). Similarly, American students seeking a global health experience in Africa or elsewhere in the "developing" world are engaged in a kind of learning experiment, in which easy access to patient bodies allows them the opportunity to test and refine their nascent clinical skills under the auspices of providing medical aid. As others have already noted, the primary beneficiaries of these short-term encounters may be North American "clinical tourists" (Wendland 2012), who find their knowledge and resumes enhanced, and not patients, who may suffer as a result of foreign students' inexperience (Crump and Sugarman 2008). In addition, like private-sector science, academic global health research benefits from the surfeit of untreated or "treatment-naïve" patients in low-income countries, which provide research subjects in numbers that cannot be duplicated in the global North. The premium placed on "baseline" blood samples by the University of California researchers described in chapter 3 is one example of this.

However, academic global health training and research are not typically profit-driven, and this remains an important difference between the kind of work undertaken by members of the CUGH and the contract research organizations described by Petryna. This leaves us with another question: if not profit, what drives these students and researchers to pursue "global health"? In my own experience, they are moved both by a sincere humanitarian desire to address suffering, and by intellectual curiosity and the opportunity to learn or produce new knowledge. These motivations, while well intentioned, should be considered in light of the long history of Northern efforts to "cure the ills" of Africans and other residents of the Southern Hemisphere through scientific medicine (Vaughan 1991). At a 2010 conference in honor of historian of Africa Steven Feierman, Nancy Rose Hunt described "extraction" and "salvation" as the two main historical modes of Northern intervention in Africa (Conference on Social Health in the New Millennium, University of Pennsylvania, April 24). I am concerned that vestiges of these colonial-era motivations may persist, albeit in attenuated forms, in today's global health involvement on the continent.

In academic global health, extraction comes in the form of scientific data production and clinical experimentality, while salvation is manifest in seemingly miraculous biomedical interventions able to snatch patients away from the jaws of death (a phenomenon most visible in HIV treatment). These twin themes are apparent in *Saving Lives: Universities Transforming Global Health*, the glossy, multipage brochure commissioned by CUGH for distribution to the U.S. Congress, where images of African women and children—the "saved"—are paired with text touting the importance of scientific inquiry and learning (Consortium of Universities for Global Health 2009). The cover of the ten-page booklet exemplifies this by featuring a large photo of an African mother holding her ailing baby, underneath the banner "Saving Lives." On the following page there is a caption describing this photo, as well as a suggestion as to how the suffering it depicts might be remedied. "A mother holds her 8-month old daughter at Hospital LeDantec in Dakar, Senegal," we are told. "The child, whose lips are blue from lack of oxygen, had pneumonia." Then, the next sentence offers up a solution: "Research conducted by Boston University investigators will lead to earlier interventions for severe pneumonia, cutting down the number of cases such as this one and saving lives." No one would dispute the need to invest global health dollars into fighting pneumonia, which kills more children worldwide than any other disease, or the need for public health research that could contribute to better treatment and prevention (UNICEF 2006). It is the positioning of North American scientists as saviors of Africans—there is no mention of Senegalese scientists in the caption—and the erasure of the power relations that structure scientific knowledge production in global health that are troubling here.

The legacy of colonial-era inequalities is an uncomfortable topic in global health, and one that the field seeks to avoid reproducing through the invocation of an ethic of "partnership." However, as I hope I have shown, the espousal of partnership—while a noble aspiration—runs the risk of obfuscating both the enduring and novel forms of inequality that shape the transnational relations of global health. This includes the dependence of Northern global health programs on easy access to the bodies of under-treated patients in (or, in the case of refugees, from) the global South, and the difficulty in envisioning how Southern clinicians and researchers might learn or practice global health. This complicated and paradoxical relationship to inequality is not usually addressed by North American actors and institutions within the field, who tend to position their activities as straightforwardly beneficial for both wealthy sponsor nations and lower-income host countries. To be fair, these programs do bring benefits to institutions in poor countries, and their presence is most often quite welcome. However, if global health wishes to truly make strides toward its ethic of equitable partnership, the field must make a more genuine effort to grapple with the unequal terrain on which it operates and which, ultimately, serves as its condition of possibility.

Conclusion

In 2011, the world marked the thirtieth anniversary of the June 5, 1981, CDC report documenting five unusual cases of *pneumocystis* pneumonia in young, previously healthy gay men in Los Angeles (CDC 1981). Traditionally, this report is viewed as the first official recognition of the disease that would come to be known as AIDS, and its publication has become a stand-in for the onset of the global epidemic. Other, less official forms of recognition came earlier—both in the United States, where gay men and their doctors started noticing inexplicable infections in the 1970s—and in central and east Africa, where doctors noticed a spike in illnesses during the late 1970s and early 1980s and people began referring to a new affliction called "slim" or "Juliana's disease" (Iliffe 2006; Thornton 2008; Garrett 1994). This unofficial recognition, however, would remain just that: unpublished, "local" knowledge lacking the imprimatur of scientific expertise. In this way, the CDC's 1981 publication marks another less recognized beginning, that of the hegemony of biomedical expertise—and American biomedical science in particular—in framing the epidemic.

Thirty years later, the AIDS epidemic and the global health science to which it gave birth are at a crossroads. In 2010, U.S. government funding for ARV programs via PEPFAR flatlined as the Obama administration's Global Health Initiative attempted to reorient the emphasis of U.S. global health funding towards maternal and child health (Sahoo 2010). In 2012, the Global Health Initiative's office closed and its work was shifted elsewhere (though the Office of the Global AIDS Coordinator, which oversees PEPFAR, remains in place; Donnelly 2012). Meanwhile, U.S. and other donations to the Global Fund to Fight AIDS, Tuberculosis and Malaria have declined, forcing the foundation to cease issuing new grants and spurring a $750 million donation by the Bill and Melinda Gates Foundation to "shore up" the Fund (McNeil 2012). Although both PEPFAR and the Global Fund voice a commitment to continue supporting treatment for those already on ARVs, public funding to expand treatment access to new patients is becoming increasingly uncertain. Some have suggested that the scaling-up of ARV access and the "golden age" of global health funding have come to a close (Ingram 2012; Rushton and Williams 2011.

At the same time, the remarkable achievements of these programs in changing the global landscape of HIV treatment should not be overlooked. By 2010, the WHO estimated that over 6.6 million people in low- and middle-income countries were receiving antiretroviral treatment—a seventeen-fold increase since 2003. Of these 6.6 million, over 5 million were in sub-Saharan Africa (WHO, UNICEF, and UNAIDS 2011, 89–90). Furthermore, improvements in therapy mean that those taking ARVs are now capable of living normal, relatively healthy life spans in which their HIV infection may never progress to AIDS. This development, along with new scientific findings suggesting the protective effect of male circumcision and the utility of antiretroviral treatment in preventing new infections, led Secretary of State Hillary Clinton to declare the possibility of an "AIDS-free generation" in the near future (McNeil 2011b). While the possibility (and the meaning) of this pronouncement are subjects of debate, it should be noted that much of the research that made Clinton's declaration possible was conducted in southern and eastern Africa, providing further evidence that the locus, if not always the control, of some of the most prominent recent findings in AIDS science is now in Africa. Moreover, even as U.S. government funding for global health rests on unsteady ground, the number of global health programs at U.S. and Canadian universities tripled between

2006 and 2011, suggesting that the enthusiasm for global health within the North American academy continues unabated (Doughton 2011). There is further proof of this in Mbarara, where plans are underway to build an 18,000 square foot public health conference and education center aimed at strengthening global health research and education at the university and in the broader region. The construction of the center, which will be a part of MUST, is being managed by the global health program at Beale's academic medical center in the United States.

These developments raise questions about where American global health science is heading, and how and whether HIV/AIDS fits into its future. They suggest, as I have tried to illustrate in this book, that the outcomes of global health science are uneven. On one hand, the AIDS epidemic and subsequent rise of "global health" have led to greater engagement between universities and medical centers in the United States and in the global South, particularly in sub-Saharan Africa. This engagement, in turn, has brought new opportunities and resources to African institutions and experts, fostered greater collaboration between African and American colleagues, and pushed AIDS science to account for the global diversity of HIV. On the other hand, global health science has brought with it a host of new inequalities, many of which trouble the field's leaders' fervent espousal of an ethic of "partnership." Some of these inequalities are visible at the level of institutions: for example, the circumvention and undercutting of African public health and educational systems by American medical schools eager to avoid local bureaucracy, or the primacy of a few, U.S.-certified African laboratories in determining the landscape of global health knowledge-making. Others are more apparent on the micro-social level of human relations, such as the tensions that arose around the Wellness Clinic's database, or Dr. Balenzi's careful conversation with me about her medical staff's desire to be compensated for their interviews. What these ongoing disparities show us is that as the field of global health strives to reduce human suffering, it must not ignore the unequal social relations of science and medicine that it can engender.

Ethnography is one means of getting at these social relations, as its rigorous contextualization of human lives forces us to understand the actions of individuals as both socially and historically produced. By examining the everyday practices of U.S. and Ugandan global health researchers as both emerging from and (sometimes) challenging a scientific landscape that is deeply geographically and economically stratified, this book represents an effort to push global health science to recognize and confront the inequalities that make it both possible and productive. For this reason, it seems appropriate to conclude by returning to ethnography to consider the question of global health's future. While I do not presume to be able to predict this future, two ethnographic vignettes from my research serve as cautionary tales.

Mbarara, 2009

In the summer of 2009, I sat on a wooden bench in the hallway of the Immune Wellness Clinic waiting for a doctor who had agreed to be interviewed for my research. My seat happened to be directly across from one of the clinic's two pharmacies. I sat facing what staff called the "OI pharmacy," two small adjoining rooms where patients went to obtain the antibiotics, antifungals, and other drugs needed to treat any HIV-related opportunistic infections (OIs) they might be suffering from. (Antiretroviral drugs were dispensed from a separate pharmacy.) There was music coming from a radio inside and a pharmacist at work in there, as well as regular traffic in and out by clinicians and other staff. The rooms had windows that faced out onto the clinic hallway, and through them I could see inside to a wall of glass-fronted cabinets filled with bottles of prescription drugs: septrin, acyclovir, fluconazole. There were also stacked cardboard boxes of more drugs waiting to be unpacked. These were each hand-labeled in magic marker with the name of the clinic "stakeholder" that had paid for them: the Ugandan Ministry of Health, and two separate PEPFAR-funded programs.

What drew my attention most, however, was a memo that was posted on the pharmacy door. Dated October 2, 2008, it was addressed to "all staff" from "management." It read:

> This is to inform all staff of this clinic and Hospital that all Drugs at the Immune Wellness Clinic are strictly for the patients Registered with the clinic. Therefore anyone who requires drugs should find a way of obtaining them elsewhere.

Later, Dr. Atuhaire and Dr. Balenzi explained the memo to me. Unlike the clinic's separate ARV pharmacy, which dispensed drugs useful only to patients with HIV, the OI pharmacy offered medicines for the treatment of all sorts of infections. Like ARVs, these drugs were purchased with monies from PEPFAR and the Global Fund (via the Ministry of Health) and provided to Wellness Clinic patients free of charge. To obtain their pills, patients simply had to hand their prescription through the window to a pharmacist and wait about five minutes for the medication to be dispensed. The pharmacist would then record the exchange on a spreadsheet called the "Drug Dispensing Sheet," which was entered into the clinic database at the end of each day.

At times, the doctors told me, patients who were not enrolled at the Wellness Clinic would attempt to obtain medications from the OI pharmacy. These were HIV-negative patients who had been seen at other clinics within the university hospital, but had been unable to fill their prescriptions at the hospital's outpatient pharmacy, which was frequently out of stock of all but the most basic drugs. Unable to afford to buy medication at the private pharmacies in town, patients who knew about the OI pharmacy would sometimes attempt to get their prescriptions filled there. This was a particularly difficult issue with "discordant" couples, Dr. Balenzi told me. "A wife with HIV may come in and get her treatment but her [HIV-negative] husband, who also needs something, can't get drugs."

Although such patients would occasionally come to the OI pharmacy in person asking for medication, more often they tried to enlist the help of a friend or relative who worked at the clinic. The memo on the door was thus intended to remind staff that providing drugs to patients not receiving HIV care was forbidden. The Wellness Clinic could not afford to provide free drugs to patients without HIV, Dr. Atuhaire told me, "because we have to give accountabilities at the end of the month. We know the number of patients we are providing care for, so we are able to make accountabilities [to donors] that we received this number of tins of septrin and we have dispensed it as follows." Nonetheless, he was sympathetic with the inequality inherent within the situation, telling me: "Two patients come to the hospital, one goes to the hospital outpatient clinic, sees a doctor, and all the medications that have been written have to be bought. The one who has gone to the same hospital but to the HIV clinic gets a prescription, and all the drugs written are provided. For free."

Seattle, 2012

In the summer of 2012, residents of and visitors to the city of Seattle were invited to have a global health experience without ever leaving the city. The "Global Health Experience" exhibit, housed just a few hundred yards from the city's iconic Space Needle, was just one of several events comprising "Global Health Month" in Seattle. The month was organized by the "Global Health Nexus," a consortium of academic, medical, philanthropic, and private research institutions in Washington state "dedicated to branding our region internationally as the nexus for global health discovery, development, and delivery" (Puget Sound Regional Council 2012). It was conceived as one of many events comprising "The Next Fifty"—a six-month celebration commemorating the fiftieth anniversary of the Seattle World's Fair. Held at the Seattle Center, an urban event space originally built to house the 1962 fair, "The Next Fifty" was intended not only to celebrate Seattle's past but also to foster "a dialogue about our future" (Seattle Center Foundation 2011). Given that it is home to the Bill and Melinda Gates Foundation,[1] the nonprofit Program for Appropriate Technology in Health (PATH), and the University of Washington's Department of Global Health, it is perhaps not surprising that Seattle's business and political leaders would promote it as a "curative global city" (Sparke 2011).

Visitors to the Global Health Experience entered the exhibit's warehouse-like space through a large doorway emblazoned with photographs of African children captioned "4 lives, 4 countries, 4 challenges to survival." Additional text promised "hands on activities—free and for the whole family." Upon entering, visitors could wind their way through four different "life lanes" each focused on a different global health challenge—cancer, diabetes, maternal health, and malaria—and profiling the ways in which Washington-based organizations and companies were working to ameliorate it.

The exhibit spaces were designed as life-size dioramas aimed at transporting visitors to impoverished settings in the global South: for example, in

---

1. Both the Global Health Nexus and Global Health Month were heavily supported by the Gates Foundation, which is headquartered across the street from the Seattle Center. The foundation is the world's largest philanthropic organization, and global health is its largest grant-making area.

the "cancer lane," set in Uganda, visitors walked through a room with "mud" walls (constructed out of plastic), filled with holes and blackened by smoke from a charcoal stove. The "malaria lane," set in Tanzania, featured a room with corrugated tin walls and furnished with a single, uncovered foam mat lying on the floor. In both cases, these stark conditions and the bare survival they evoked were juxtaposed with photos and text that detailed the efforts of Seattle area organizations to diagnose, treat, or prevent such diseases. The Ugandan cancer exhibit, for example, described "*care*HPV™," a technology "co-developed by PATH" and aimed at diagnosing the human papilloma virus, which is linked to cervical cancer. (The test's other developer, a multinational medical diagnostics corporation called Quiagen, was not mentioned in the exhibit.) The diabetes exhibit, in turn, promoted the "HumanPen Memoir™," an insulin-delivery device designed to help patients remember their injections. The device was developed by the pharmaceutical firm Eli Lilly and the research and development organization Battelle, which has major offices in western Washington state.

In addition to the four disease-specific "life lanes," the Global Health Experience also devoted a large area to clean water and sanitation efforts—featuring water-purification and latrine technologies developed by Seattle-area groups—and an additional section simply titled "Other Cool Technologies." This area displayed inventions ranging from "Partopants," a low-tech birth simulator designed to train birth attendants in the management of obstetric emergencies (designed at the University of Washington), to "Ultra Rice," a manufactured "grain" made from rice flour and fortified with micronutrients developed by PATH and the private U.S. company Bon Dente International. As visitors left the exhibit space, they were encouraged to visit the "Pathways to Global Health" exhibition in a neighboring building, where they could learn about local education and career options in global health.

"We Are Somewhere"

It is easy to see the ways in which the spaces in these two vignettes are divergent. Located half a world away from one another, Mbarara's Immune Wellness Clinic and Seattle's Global Health Experience not only occupy separate continents but also serve separate purposes, one curative and one promotional. More importantly, they differ profoundly in their access to resources and proximity to bodily suffering. Yet I would argue that these sites actually have quite a bit to say to one another.

First, both places raise questions about the role of HIV/AIDS in global health. The notice on the door of the Wellness Clinic's OI pharmacy is a mundane yet profound marker of how HIV/AIDS has dominated global health funding and actions, often at the expense of other, less spectacular but equally lethal illnesses. The result, as many critics have noted, is an "AIDS exceptionalism" within global health that offers state-of-the-art care to those suffering from HIV (and to some extent, TB and malaria), but leaves other diseases and broader public health concerns unaddressed (Ingram 2012; Biehl 2007; Garrett 2007).[2] Global health research has mirrored this uneven attention, focusing primarily on the "big three" of AIDS, TB, and malaria. For this reason, the absence of HIV/AIDS from the Global Health Experience exhibit is noteworthy. The exhibit's limited attention to infectious disease and its highlighting of chronic illnesses (cancer, diabetes) often thought of as "first-world" diseases suggests a broadening of the scope of global health and a growing recognition of illnesses and concerns other than HIV. While the story of the Wellness Clinic pharmacy exemplifies what happens to medical care when global health is limited to a "pharmaceuticalized" response to AIDS, the Seattle exhibit suggests a technology-driven response to global health in which HIV/AIDS is no longer a primary concern.

Secondly, these sites are similar in their demonstration of an oft-noted and worrisome trend in global health: the turn away from public health. In Mbarara, a visit to the public hospital's outpatient pharmacy—stocked by the Ministry of Health—confirmed what Dr. Atuhaire had described. Although the pharmacy was able to provide patients with "basic" drugs like antimalarials, some antibiotics, and Panadol (acetaminophen), the pharmacist on duty told me that the drug supply varied from month to month, and that they regularly suffered from stock-outs. For "complicated" drugs "like Keflex" (a branded antibiotic), patients were often sent to private pharmacies in town, where they had to purchase the medications themselves.

---

2. Exceptionalism shaped domestic responses to the AIDS epidemic within the United States as well (Bayer 1999; Casarett and Lantos 1998; Crane, Quirk, and Van der Straten 2002).

Hypertension and diabetes patients were particularly difficult to treat, he said, as insulin and blood pressure medications were not available through the Ministry and often too expensive for patients to buy in town. No wonder, then, that hospital patients would sometimes find their way to the well-stocked, internationally-funded OI pharmacy at the Wellness Clinic in hopes that they might find what they needed.

If African public health has been hollowed out in Mbarara it is nonetheless still visible in the form of the doctors, nurses, and pharmacists who continue to treat patients under the hospital's conditions of "normal emergency" (Feierman 2011). But in the "Global Health Experience" offered up to visitors in Seattle, African government health systems have been almost completely erased. Instead, global health is framed as a series of technical problems offering new market niches for American ingenuity and public-private product development. Scholars have rightly criticized this "private turn" in global health governance as marginalizing state systems and traditional international bodies such as the WHO while promoting a technical approach to global health that sidelines basic public health (Rushton and Williams 2011; Benatar 2005; Lakoff 2010).[3] This is not to say that there is no room for useful technology development in global health; ARVs have proven as much. But when a patented insulin-delivery pen is promoted as an adherence-enhancing device for diabetics in places where insulin is not available via the public sector, it is difficult not to view this action as predatory.

It is not only African public health that is absent from the "Global Health Experience"—it is also African expertise. This brings me to my final point: in order to truly enact the ethic of partnership it espouses, global health science must account for the social relations of knowledge production it engenders. Moreover, it must strive to make these social relations of science more equitable just as it aims to make health more equal. My concluding ethnographic snapshots reveal very different paths in this regard. Other than a brief mention of the Uganda Cancer Institute (which has a

---

3. The Gates Foundation, which has been criticized for its emphasis on top-down technology development and quantifiable outcomes over qualitative and collaborative improvements in basic public health, has been particularly influential in promoting technology-driven approaches to global health due to its vast wealth and substantial scientific and political influence (Birn 2005; McCoy et al. 2009).

partnership with the Fred Hutchison Center for Cancer Research in Seattle), the Seattle exhibit's displays say very little about knowledge production by African (or Asian, or Latin American) researchers. Rather, the primary representation of the global South is one of destitution and often ignorance. Africa is once again a place in need of salvation by Western intervention. The life-size dioramas of mud shacks and threadbare existence are in many ways a return to the "dirty water and mud roads" imagery of Africa that dominated the debates over global ARV access that I described in chapter 1, a key difference being that now these impoverished conditions are envisioned not as a barrier to high-tech medicine, but as a market niche for (Western-developed) technologies designed specifically for "low-resource settings." This brings us full circle: underdevelopment has been transformed from a barrier to treatment into a medical technologies market opportunity. But the social relations of science, in which "authorities in rich countries [debate] what is to be done for (or to) the poor" have remained the same (Feierman 2011, 190).

By contrast, the Wellness Clinic, despite its ongoing inequalities, provides an important counter to the Seattle exhibit's vision of global health science. At the clinic, Ugandan doctors and researchers are indispensible to the production of scientific knowledge about HIV and AIDS. Dr. Beale's research endeavors have been very successful, both in the scientific findings they have produced and in the resources they have brought to the clinic, and his career has advanced substantially as a result. None of this would have been possible without collaborators like Dr. Atuhaire, whose methodical clinical record keeping served as the foundation upon which the transnational scientific collaboration could be built. Moreover, it was Atuhaire's colleagues at the Wellness Clinic who ultimately enabled its transformation from a "local" clinic into a "global" research site by—sometimes reluctantly—serving as gatherers of clinical data on the patients under their care. As I hope this book has shown, the outcomes of this transformation— and others like it across Africa—have been uneven. Without a doubt, the transnational scientific communities being forged in Mbarara and elsewhere have yielded important scientific insight into HIV/AIDS and other health problems facing poor countries, as well as valuable intellectual and professional opportunities for the aspiring Ugandan researchers with the good fortune to become, in the words of Dr. Katabira, "attached to someone" like Dr. Beale. At the same time, the tensions over the meaning and purpose of the Wellness Clinic database and other research conducted on the premises (including my own) should remind us that the symbiotic relationship this work suggests is at best a lopsided one.

The spaces of global health science are spaces of "friction," where the work of studying and redressing global health inequalities often generates new forms of inclusion and exclusion. At the Wellness Clinic, these frictions—although challenging—were also productive in that they forced difficult but important conversations about who benefits from international research, and the unequal relationships of power and economics that underlie collaborations between U.S. and African scientists. In contrast to the abject picture of Africa presented in the Seattle exhibit, the work being done by the international community of doctors and researchers at the Wellness Clinic and medical school repudiates the imaginary of Africa as "down to the dogs" by affirming, as one Mbarara doctor insisted, that "we are somewhere." Their stories also highlight the hard work involved in working towards "true partnership" across steep inequalities, and reveal the uncomfortable mix of preventable suffering and scientific productivity that characterize global health. However uncomfortable, this recognition should serve as a critique, but not a condemnation, of global health. It is only through confronting the ways in which global health values inequality that we can work towards building a more equal global health science.

REFERENCES

HIV type determines how fast you die. *The New Vision.* March 1, 2006.

Immunocompromised homosexuals [editorial]. 1981. *The Lancet* 2 (8259): 1325–6.

Adams, Vincanne. 2010a. Against global health? Arbitrating science, non-science, and nonsense through health. In *Against health: How health became the new morality*, ed. Jonathan Metzl and Anna Kirkland, 40–60. New York: New York University Press.

———. 2010b. Evidence-based global public health: Subjects, profits, erasures. Paper presented at "When People Come First: Anthropology and Social Innovation in the Field of Global Health" Conference, Princeton University. March 11–13.

———. 2002. Randomized controlled crime: Postcolonial studies in alternative medicine research. *Social Studies of Science* 32 (5–6): 659–90.

Adje-Toure, C., B. Celestin, D. Hanson, T. H. Roels, K. Hertogs, B. Larder, F. Diomande, et al. 2003. Prevalence of genotypic and phenotypic HIV-1 drug-resistant strains among patients who have rebound in viral load while receiving antiretroviral therapy in the UNAIDS-drug access initiative in Abidjan, Cote d'Ivoire. *AIDS (London, England)* 17 Suppl 3 (Jul): S23–9.

AfriCASO (African Council of AIDS Service Organizations). 2000. *The Nairobi Declaration: An African appeal for an AIDS vaccine.* Nairobi, Kenya. June 14.

AIDS Vaccine Advocacy Coalition (AVAC). 2005. *AIDS vaccines at the crossroads.* Accessed November 13, 2008, http://www.avac.org/pdf/reports/AVAC_Report_2005.pdf.

Allen, Tim. 1991. The quest for therapy in Moyo district. In *Changing Uganda: The dilemmas of structural adjustment and revolutionary change,* ed. H. B. Hansen and M. Twaddle, 149–161. London: James Currey.

Altman, Dennis. 1988. Legitimation through disaster: AIDS and the gay movement. In *AIDS: The burdens of history,* ed. E. Fee and D. Fox, 301–315. Berkeley: University of California Press.

Altman, Lawrence. 1998. Parts of Africa showing H.I.V. in 1 in 4 adults. *New York Times,* Jun 24.

Anderson, Warwick. 2008. *The collectors of lost souls: Turning kuru scientists into whitemen.* Baltimore: Johns Hopkins University Press.

———. 2002. Postcolonial technoscience. *Social Studies of Science* 32 (5–6): 643–58.

Anderson, Warwick, and Vincanne Adams. 2008. Pramoedya's chickens: Postcolonial studies of technoscience. In *The handbook of science and technology studies,* ed. E. J. Hackett, O. Amsterdamska, M. Lynch and J. Wajcman. 3rd ed. Cambridge, MA: MIT Press.

Atlas, A, F. Granath, A. Lindstrom, K. Lidman, S. Lindback, and A. Alaeus. 2005. Impact of HIV type 1 genetic subtype on the outcome of antiretroviral therapy. *AIDS Research and Human Retroviruses* 21 (3) (Mar): 221–7.

AVERT. 2008. PEPFAR prime partners in fiscal year 2007. Accessed June 22, 2010, www.avert.org/media/pdfs/pepfar-partners07.pdf.

Bajunirwe, Francis. 2011. Feasibility and effectiveness of a mobile antiretroviral pharmacy in rural Uganda. Paper presented at Global Health Week 2011: Northwestern in the World, Northwestern University. April 8.

Bangsberg, D. R., E. D. Charlebois, R. M. Grant, M. Holodniy, S. G. Deeks, S. Perry, K. N. Conroy, et al. 2003. High levels of adherence do not prevent accumulation of HIV drug resistance mutations. *AIDS (London, England)* 17 (13) (Sep 5): 1925–32.

Bangsberg, D. R., and S. G. Deeks. 2002. Is average adherence to HIV antiretroviral therapy enough? *Journal of General Internal Medicine: Official Journal of the Society for Research and Education in Primary Care Internal Medicine* 17 (10) (Oct): 812–3.

Bangsberg, D. R., A. R. Moss, and S. G. Deeks. 2004. Paradoxes of adherence and drug resistance to HIV antiretroviral therapy. *The Journal of Antimicrobial Chemotherapy* 53 (5) (May): 696–9.

Barbanel, Josh. 1991. Rise in tuberculosis forces review of dated methods. *New York Times.* July 7.

Barbour, J. D., T. Wrin, R. M. Grant, J. N. Martin, M. R. Segal, C. J. Petropoulos, and S. G. Deeks. 2002. Evolution of phenotypic drug susceptibility and viral replication capacity during long-term virologic failure of protease inhibitor therapy in human immunodeficiency virus-infected adults. *Journal of Virology* 76 (21) (Nov): 11104–12.

Baxter, Daniel. 1997. Casting off the 'unreliable' AIDS patient. *New York Times,* Mar 6.

Bayer, R. 1999. Clinical progress and the future of HIV exceptionalism. *Archives of Internal Medicine* 159 (10) (May 24): 1042–8.

Bayer, R., and J. Stryker. 1997. Ethical challenges posed by clinical progress in AIDS. *American Journal of Public Health* 87 (10) (Oct): 1599–602.

Behrman, Greg. 2004. *The invisible people.* New York: Free Press.

Belkin, Lisa. 1991. Top TB peril: Not taking the medicine. *New York Times,* November 18.

Benatar, S. R. 2005. Moral imagination: The missing component in global health. *PLoS Medicine* 2 (12) (Dec): e400.

Biehl, Joao. 2007. *Will to live: AIDS therapies and the politics of survival.* Princeton: Princeton University Press.

Birn, A. E. 2005. Gates's grandest challenge: Transcending technology as public health ideology. *Lancet* 366 (9484) (Aug 6–12): 514–9.

Biruk, Crystal. 2012. Seeing like a research project: Producing "high quality" data in AIDS research in Malawi. *Medical Anthropology* 31(4): 347–366.

Birungi, Harriet. 1998. Injections and self-help: Risk and trust in Ugandan health care. *Social Science and Medicine* 47 (10): 1455–62.

Bledsoe, Caroline. 2002. *Contingent lives: Fertility, time, and aging in west Africa.* Chicago: University of Chicago Press.

Blick, G., R. M. Kagan, E. Coakley, C. Petropoulos, L. Maroldo, P. Greiger-Zanlungo, S. Gretz, and T. Garton. 2007. The probable source of both the primary multidrug-resistant (MDR) HIV-1 strain found in a patient with rapid progression to AIDS and a second recombinant MDR strain found in a chronically HIV-1–infected patient. *Journal of Infectious Diseases* 195(May1): 1250–9.

Bond, George C., and Joan Vincent. 1991. Living on the edge: Changing social structures in the context of AIDS. In *Changing Uganda: The dilemmas of structural adjustment and revolutionary change,* ed. H. B. Hansen and M. Twaddle, 113–130. London: James Currey.

Booth, C. L., and A. M. Geretti. 2007. Prevalence and determinants of transmitted antiretroviral drug resistance in HIV-1 infection. *The Journal of Antimicrobial Chemotherapy* 59 (6) (Jun): 1047–56.

Bornstein, Erica. 2010. The value of orphans. In *Forces of compassion: Humanitarianism between ethics and politics,* ed. Peter Redfield and Erica Bornstein, 123–148. Santa Fe: School for Advanced Research Press.

Bourgois, Philippe, Mark Lettiere, and James Quesada. 1997. Social misery and the sanctions of substance abuse: Confronting HIV risk among homeless heroin addicts in San Francisco. *Social Problems* 44 (2): 155–73.

Bourgois, Philippe, and Jeffrey Schonberg. 2009. *Righteous dopefiend.* Berkeley: University of California Press.

Boyer, Dominic. 2008. Thinking through the anthropology of experts. *Anthropology in Action* 15 (2): 38–46.

Brada, B. 2011a. Botswana as a living experiment. PhD diss., University of Chicago.

———. 2011b. "Not *here*": Making the spaces and subjects of global health in Botswana. *Culture, Medicine, and Psychiatry* 35 (2): 285–312.

Braitstein, P., M. W. Brinkhof, F. Dabis, M. Schechter, A. Boulle, P. Miotti, R. Wood, et al. 2006. Mortality of HIV-1-infected patients in the first year of antiretroviral therapy: Comparison between low-income and high-income countries. *The Lancet* 367 (9513) (Mar 11): 817–24.

Brenner, B. G. 2007. Resistance and viral subtypes: How important are the differences and why do they occur? *Current Opinion in HIV and AIDS* 2 (2) (Mar): 94–102.

Briggs, Charles, and Clara Mantini-Briggs. 2003. *Stories in the time of cholera.* Berkeley: University of California Press.

Brower, V. 2005. New superbug or tempest in a teapot? *EMBO Reports* 6(6): 502–504.

Brown, David. 2008. For a global generation, public health is a hot field. *Washington Post,* Sept. 19.

Brown, T. M., M. Cueto, and E. Fee. 2006. The World Health Organization and the transition from "international" to "global" public health. *American Journal of Public Health* 96 (1) (Jan): 62–72.

Bunyavanich, S., and R. B. Walkup. 2001. U.S. public health leaders shift toward a new paradigm of global health. *American Journal of Public Health* 91 (10) (Oct): 1556–8.

Byakika-Tusiime, J., J. H. Oyugi, W. A. Tumwikirize, E. T. Katabira, P.E. Mugyenyi, and D. R. Bangsberg. 2005. Adherence to HIV antiretroviral therapy in HIV+ Ugandan patients purchasing therapy. *International Journal of STD & AIDS* 16: 38–41.

Carpenter, Elise Audrey. 2010. The invisible bureaucrat in Botswana's HIV drug therapy program. Paper presented at Social Health in the New Millennium: A Conference in Honor of Steven Feierman, University of Pennsylvania. April 23.

———. 2008. The social practice of HIV drug therapy in Botswana, 2002–2004: Experts, bureaucrats, and health care providers. PhD diss., University of Pennsylvania.

Casarett, D. J., and J. D. Lantos. 1998. Have we treated AIDS too well? Rationing and the future of AIDS exceptionalism. *Annals of Internal Medicine* 128 (9) (May 1): 756–9.

CDC (Centers for Disease Control and Prevention). 1992. 1993 revised classification system for HIV infection and expanded surveillance case definition for AIDS among adolescents and adults. *Morbidity and Mortality Weekly Report* 41 (RR–17). Dec 18.

———. 1982. Current trends update on acquired immune deficiency syndrome (AIDS)—United States. *Morbidity and Mortality Weekly Report* 31 (7): 507–8. Sept 24.

———. 1981. *Pneumocystis* pnuemonia—Los Angeles. *Morbidity and Mortality Weekly Report* 30 (21): 1–3. June 5.

———. 1996. Update: Trends in AIDS incidence—United States 1996. *Morbidity and Mortality Weekly Report* 46 (37): 861–7.

Chakrabarty, Dipesh. 2000. Provincializing Europe: Postcolonial thought and historical difference.

Chesney, M. 2003. Adherence to HAART regimens. *AIDS Patient Care and STDs* 17 (4) (Apr): 169–77.

Chigwedere, P., G. R. Seage, S. Gruskin, T. H. Lee, and M. Essex. 2008. Estimating the lost benefits of antiretroviral drug use in South Africa. *Journal of Acquired Immune Deficiency Syndromes (1999)* 49 (4) (Dec 1): 410–5.

City of New York. 2005. New York City resident diagnosed with rare strain of multidrug resistant HIV that rapidly progresses to AIDS. Department of Health and Mental Hygiene, Feb 11. Accessed February 1, 2013, http://www.nyc.gov/html/doh/html/pr/pr016-05.shtml.

Clarke, Adele, and Joan Fujimura. 1992. What tools? Which jobs? Why right? In *The right tools for the job: At work in the 20th century life sciences,* ed. Adele Clarke, Joan Fujimura. Princeton: Princeton University Press.

Clarke, Adele, and Susan Leigh Star. 2003. Symbolic interactionist science, technology, information, and medicine studies. In *Handbook of symbolic interactionism,* ed. Larry Reynolds, Nancy J. Herman-Kinney. Walnut Creek, CA: Alta Mira Press.

Cohen, J. 2005. Experts Question Danger of 'AIDS Superbug.' *Science* 307(5713): 1185.

College of American Pathologists. 2012. Accredited laboratory directory. Accessed September 10, 2012, http://www.cap.org/apps/cap.portal?_nfpb=true&_pageLabel= accrlabsearch_page.

Collins, Huntly. 1996. Among the poor, battling the odds: The rigid regimen of the new drugs requires more discipline than many can muster. *Philadelphia Inquirer*, Dec 30.

Comaroff, Jean. 2007. Beyond bare life: AIDS, (bio)politics, and the neoliberal order. *Public Culture* 19 (1): 197–219.

Conference on Retroviruses and Opportunistic Infections (CROI). 2005. Special Symposium: Transmitted HIV-1 Drug Resistance and Rapid Disease Progression. Boston, MA. Feb 24.

Consortium of Universities for Global Health. Membership information and application. 2012. Accessed January 19, 2012, http://www.cugh.org/?q=membership/join.

———. *Saving lives: Universities transforming global health*. Consortium of Universities for Global Health, 2009.

———. 2008. *Meeting report: University Consortium for Global Health inaugural meeting*. Accessed May 13, 2010, http://www.cugh.org/sites/default/files/inaugural-meeting -report.pdf.

Cooper, Helene, Rachel Zimmerman, and Laurie McGinley. 2001. Patents pending: AIDS epidemic traps drug firms in a vise. *Wall Street Journal*, March 2.

Cooper, Melissa. 2007. Life, autopoesis, debt: Inventing the bioeconomy. *Distinktion: Scandanavian Journal of Social Theory* 14: 25–43.

Cornell University Division of Nutritional Sciences. 2012. Field experience. Accessed September 8, 2012, http://www.human.cornell.edu/che/DNS/globalhealth/under graduate/field.cfm.

Craddock, Susan. 2007. Market incentives, human lives, and AIDS vaccines. *Social Science and Medicine* 64: 1042–56.

Crane, Johanna T. 2010a. Adverse events and placebo effects: African scientists, HIV, and ethics in the "global health sciences." *Social Studies of Science* 40 (6): 843–70.

———. 2010b. Scrambling for Africa? Universities and global health. *Lancet* 377 (Nov): 1113.

———. 2007. The molecularization of forgiveness: Race, blame, and antiretroviral adherence. Paper presented at the Annual Meeting of the American Anthropological Association. Washington, D.C., November 28.

Crane, J.T., A. Kawuma, J.H. Oyugi, J.T. Byakika, A. Moss, P. Bourgois, and D. R. Bangsberg. 2006. The price of adherence: Qualitative findings from HIV positive individuals purchasing fixed-dose combination generic HIV antiretroviral therapy in Kampala, Uganda. *AIDS and Behavior* 10(4): 437–442.

Crane, Johanna T., Kathleen Quirk, and Ariane Van der Straten. 2002. 'Come back when you're dying:' the commodification of AIDS among California's urban poor. *Social Science and Medicine* 55 (7): 1115–27.

Crimp, Douglas, and Adam Rolston. 1990. *AIDS demographics*. San Francisco: Bay Press.

Crump, J. A., and J. Sugarman. 2008. Ethical considerations for short-term experiences by trainees in global health. *JAMA: The Journal of the American Medical Association* 300 (12) (Sep 24): 1456–8.

De Laet, Marianne, ed. 2002. *Research in science and technology studies: Knowledge and technology transfer.* Greenwich, CT and London: JAI Press.

De Laet, Marianne, and Annemarie Mol. 2000. The Zimbabwe bush pump: Mechanics of a fluid technology. *Social Studies of Science* 30: 225–63.

Deeks, S. G., J. D. Barbour, J. N. Martin, M. S. Swanson, and R. M. Grant. 2000. Sustained CD4+ T cell response after virologic failure of protease inhibitor-based regimens in patients with human immunodeficiency virus infection. *The Journal of Infectious Diseases* 181 (3) (Mar): 946–53.

DHHS (U.S. Department of Health and Human Services). 2003. *Guidelines for the use of antiretroviral agents in HIV-1 infected adults and adolescents.* Accessed June 8, 2007, http://*AIDSinfo*.nih.gov.

Dodge, Cole P., and Paul D. Wiebe, ed. 1985. *Crisis in Uganda: The breakdown of health services.* Oxford: Pergemon Press.

Donnelly, John. 2012. Obama administration closes global health initiative office. *Global Post,* July 3. Accessed September 9, 2012, http://www.globalpost.com/dispatches/globalpost-blogs/global-pulse/obama-administration-closes-global-health-initiative-office.

———. 2001. Prevention urged in AIDS fight. *Boston Globe*, June 7.

Doughton, Sandi. 2011. UW students, faculty flock to global health program. *Seattle Times,* April 24.

Duke Global Health Institute. 2012. Medical students: Get involved in global health. Accessed September 6, 2012, http://globalhealth.duke.edu/dghi-fieldwork/students-in-the-field/individual-projects/medical-students-get-involved-in-global-health.

Duke University School of Medicine. 2012. Third year: Global health study program. Accessed September 8, 2012, http://thirdyear.mc.duke.edu/modules/dukepeople/index.php?eid=179.

Edney, Michael. 1997. *Mapping an empire: The geographical construction of British India, 1765–1843.* Chicago: University of Chicago Press.

Edozien, Frankie. 2005. New AIDS super bug: Nightmare strain shows up in city. *New York Post*, February 12.

El-Sadr, Waafa, Kenneth H. Mayer, and Sally L. Hodder. 2010. AIDS in America: Forgotten but not gone. *New England Journal of Medicine* 362 (11): 967–70.

Epstein, Elaine. 2003. *State of Denial*, DVD. Lovett Productions. South Africa/USA: California Newsreel. 83 min.

Epstein, Helen. 2007. *The invisible cure: Africa, the West, and the fight against AIDS.* New York: Farrar, Straus and Giroux.

Epstein, Steven. 1996. *Impure science: AIDS, activism, and the politics of knowledge.* Berkeley: University of California Press.

Fantini, Bernardino. 1991. Social and biological origins of the AIDS pandemic. In *AIDS and the historian: Proceedings of a conference at the National Institutes of Health 20–21, March 1989,* ed. Victoria Harden and Guenter Risse, 52–56. Bethesda, MD: National Institutes of Health.

Farmer, Paul. 2003. *Pathologies of power: Health, human rights, and the new war on the poor.* Berkeley: University of California Press.

———. 1999. *Infections and inequalities: The modern plagues*. Berkeley: University of California Press.

———. 1997. On suffering and structural violence: A view from below. In *Social suffering*, ed. A. Kleinman, V. Das and M. Lock, 261–284. Berkeley: University of California Press.

———. 1992. *AIDS and accusation: Haiti and the geography of blame*. Berkeley: University of California Press.

Farmer, Paul, and Arthur Kleinman. 1989. AIDS as human suffering. *Daedalus* 118 (2): 135–60.

Fassin, Didier. 2010a. *Noli me tangere*: The moral untouchability of humanitarianism. In *Forces of compassion: Humanitarianism between ethics and politics*, ed. Peter Redfield and Erica Bornstein, 35–52. Santa Fe: School for Advanced Research Press.

———. 2010b. Moral commitments and ethical dilemmas of humanitarianism. In *In the name of humanity: The government of threat and care*, ed. Ilana Feldman and Miriam Ticktin, 238–255. Durham: Duke University Press.

———. 2007. *When bodies remember: Experiences and politics of AIDS in South Africa*. Berkeley: University of California Press.

———. 2003. The embodiment of inequality. AIDS as a social condition and the historical experience in South Africa. *EMBO Reports* 4 Spec No (Jun): S4–9.

Feierman, Steven. 2011. When physicians meet: Local medical knowledge and global public goods. In *Evidence, ethos, and experiment: The anthropology and history of medical research in Africa*, ed. P. W. Geissler and S. Molyneux. New York: Berghahn Books.

Feierman, Steven, and John Janzen, ed. 1992. *The social basis of health and healing in Africa*. Berkeley and Los Angeles: University of California Press.

Ferguson, James. 2006. *Global shadows: Africa in the neoliberal world order*. Durham: Duke University Press.

———. 1994. *The anti-politics machine: "Development," depoliticization, and bureaucratic power in Lesotho*. Minneapolis: University of Minnesota Press.

Fleury, H. J., T. Toni, N. T. Lan, P. V. Hung, A. Deshpande, P. Recordon-Pinson, S. Boucher, et al. 2006. Susceptibility to antiretroviral drugs of CRF01_AE, CRF02_AG, and subtype C viruses from untreated patients of Africa and Asia: Comparative genotypic and phenotypic data. *AIDS Research and Human Retroviruses* 22 (4) (Apr): 357–66.

Foley, Ellen. 2010. *Your pocket is what cures you: The politics of health in Senegal*. Piscataway: Rutgers University Press.

Foucault, Michel. 1978. *The history of sexuality, vol. 1*. New York: Random House.

Fullwiley, Duana. 2011. *The encultured gene: Sickle cell health politics and biological difference in West Africa*. Princeton: Princeton University Press.

———. 2002. Life, ethics, and sickle-cell anemia: A single-gene disorder in a contingent world. PhD diss., University of California, Berkeley.

Galel, S. A., J. D. Lifson, and E. G. Engleman. 1995. Prevention of AIDS transmission through screening of the blood supply. *Annual Review of Immunology* 13: 201–27.

Gallo, R. C. 2002. Historical essay: The early years of HIV/AIDS. *Science* 298 (5599) (Nov 29): 1728–30.

Garrett, Laurie. 2007. The challenge of global health. *Foreign Affairs* 86 (14): 38.

————. 2001. HIV drugs losing power for many. *San Francisco Chronicle*, Dec 18.

————. 1994. *The coming plague: Newly emerging diseases in a world out of balance*. New York: Farrar, Straus, and Giroux.

Geissler, P. W. 2011. Transport to where? *Journal of Cultural Economy* 4 (1): 45–64.

Geissler, P. W., A. Kelly, B. Imoukhuede, and R. Pool. 2008. 'He is now like a brother, I can even give him some blood'—relational ethics and material exchanges in a malaria vaccine 'trial community' in The Gambia. *Social Science & Medicine (1982)* 67 (5) (Sep): 696–707.

Geissler, P.W., and Catherine Molyneux. 2011. *Evidence, ethos and experiment: The anthropology and history of medical research in Africa*. New York: Berghahn Books.

Geretti, A. M. 2006. HIV-1 subtypes: Epidemiology and significance for HIV management. *Current Opinion in Infectious Diseases* 19 (1) (Feb): 1–7.

Gerrets, Rene. 2010. The politics of 'partnership' in malaria research and control: A bottom-up look from a Tanzanian field site. Paper presented at the London School of Hygiene and Tropical Medicine, Medical Anthropology Seminar. Feb 23.

————. 2009. Globalizing international health: The cultural politics of 'partnership' in Tanzanian malaria control. PhD diss., New York University.

Gieryn, Thomas F. 1999. *Cultural boundaries of science: Credibility on the line*. Chicago: University of Chicago Press.

Gilbert, Hannah. 2009. Spinning blood into gold: Science, sex work, and HIV-2 in Senegal. PhD diss., McGill University.

Gilbert, Hannah. 2005. The ethnography of HIV clinical research in West Africa: Contributions of historical and science studies perspectives. Paper presented at Locating the Field: The Ethnography of Medical Research in Africa, Kilifi, Kenya. December 5–9.

Grady, Denise. 2001. Generic medicine for AIDS raises new set of concerns. *New York Times*, April 24.

Groth, Paul Erling. 1994. *Living downtown: The history of residential hotels in the United States*. Berkeley: University of California Press.

Gupta, R. K., M. R. Jordan, B. J. Sultan, A. Hill, D. H. J. Davis et al. 2012. Global trends in antiretroviral resistance in treatment-naïve individuals with HIV after rollout of antiretroviral treatment in resource-limited settings: A global collaborative study and meta-regression analysis. *The Lancet* 380(9849): 1250–1258.

Hacking, Ian. 1999. Making up people. In *The science studies reader,* ed. Mario Biagioli, 161–171. New York: Routledge.

Hahn, B. H., G. M. Shaw, S. K. Arya, M. Popovic, R. C. Gallo, and F. Wong-Staal. 1984. Molecular cloning and characterization of the HTLV-III virus associated with AIDS. *Nature* 312 (5990) (Nov 8–14): 166–9.

Hamdy, Sherine. 2012. *Our bodies belong to god: Organ transplants, Islam, and the struggle for human dignity in Egypt*. Berkeley: University of California Press.

Haraway, Donna. 1997. *Modest_Witness@Second_Millenium.FemaleMan©_Meets_ OncoMouse™: Feminism and technoscience*. New York: Routledge.

————. 1991. *Simians, cyborgs, and women: The reinvention of nature*. New York: Routledge.

Harden, Victoria. 1991. The biomedical response to AIDS in historical perspective. In *AIDS and the historian: Proceedings of a conference at the National Institutes of Health 20–21, March 1989,* ed. Victoria Harden and Guenter Risse, 36–40. Bethesda, MD: National Institutes of Health.

Harding, Sandra. 1998. *Is science multicultural? Postcolonialisms, feminisms, and epistemologies.* Bloomington: Indiana University Press.

Harding, Sandra. 1991. *Whose science? Whose knowledge? Thinking from women's lives.* Ithaca: Cornell University Press.

Harper, Ian. 2010. Extreme condition, extreme measures? Compliance, drug resistance, and the control of tuberculosis. *Anthropology & Medicine* 17 (2): 201–14.

Harries, A. D, D. S. Nyangulu, N. J. Hargreaves, O. Kaluwa, and F. M. Salaniponi. 2001. Preventing antiretroviral anarchy in sub-Saharan Africa. *Lancet* 358 (9279) (Aug 4): 410–4.

Hayden, Cori. 2003. *When nature goes public: The making and unmaking of bioprospecting in Mexico.* Princeton: Princeton University Press.

Heim, Kristi. 2010. Global health envisioned as city's next hot industry. *Seattle Times,* Feb. 25.

Helmreich, Stefan. 2008. Species of biocapital. *Science as Culture* 17 (4): 463–78.

Hodžić, Saida. 2006. Feeling human: Why emotions make development work in Ghana. Paper presented at American Anthropological Association annual meeting, Atlanta, Georgia.

Holguín, A., E. Ramirez de Arellano, P. Rivas, and V. Soriano. 2006. Efficacy of antiretroviral therapy in individuals infected with HIV-1 non-B subtypes. *AIDS Reviews* 8 (2) (Apr–Jun): 98–107.

Honigsbaum, Mark. 2005. West side story: A tale of unprotected sex which could be link to new HIV superbug. *The Guardian,* March 26.

Horton, R. 2000. African AIDS beyond Mbeki: Tripping into anarchy. *Lancet* 356 (9241) (Nov 4): 1541–2.

Hunt, Nancy Rose. 1999. *A colonial lexicon: Of birth ritual, medicalization, and mobility in the Congo.* Durham and London: Duke University Press.

Hunter, Mark. 2010. *Love in the time of AIDS: Inequality, gender, and rights in South Africa.* Bloomington: Indiana University Press.

Iliffe, John. 2002. *East African doctors: A history of the modern profession.* Kampala: Fountain Publishers.

———. 2006. *The African AIDS epidemic: A history.* Oxford: James Currey Ltd.

Ingram, Alan. 2012. After the exception: HIV/AIDS beyond salvation and scarcity. *Antipode.* August 8 2012]. Doi: 10.1111/j.1467-8330.2012.01008.x

Jacobs, Andrew. 1997. The diagnosis: HIV-positive. *New York Times,* Feb 2.

Janes, Craig, and Kitty Corbett. 2009. Anthropology and global health. *Annual Review of Anthropology* 38: 167–83.

Janzen, John. 1982. *The quest for therapy: Medical pluralism in lower Zaire.* Berkeley: University of California Press.

Jeffreys, R. 2005. Multidrug-resistant, dual-tropic HIV-1 and rapid progression. *The Lancet* 365(9475): 1923; author reply 1924.

Jülg, B., and F. D. Goebel. 2005. HIV genetic diversity: Any implications for drug resistance? *Infection* 33 (4) (Aug): 299–301.

Kahn, Joseph. 2001. Rich nations consider fund of billions to fight AIDS. *New York Times*. April 29.

Kahn, Patricia, ed. 2005. *AIDS vaccine handbook: Global perspectives*. New York: AIDS Vaccine Advocacy Coalition.

Kahn, Patricia. 2003. Do clades matter for HIV vaccines? *International AIDS Vaccine Initiative Report* (May/August). Accessed June 10, 2007, http://www.aegis.com/pubs /iavi/2003/IAVI2003-0501.html.

Kaleebu, P. 2005. HIV trials in Uganda. In *AIDS vaccine handbook: Global perspectives,* ed. Patricia Kahn, 145–152. New York: AIDS Vaccine Advocacy Coalition.

Kalipeni, E., S. Craddock, J. R. Oppong, and J. Ghosh, ed. 2003. *HIV and AIDS in Africa: Beyond epidemiology*. Malden, MA: Blackwell.

Kalofonos, Ippolytos. 2010. "All I eat is ARVs": The paradox of AIDS treatment interventions in central Mozambique. *Medical Anthropology Quarterly* 24 (3): 363–380.

Kamradt, T., D. Niese, and F. Vogel. 1985. Slim disease (AIDS). *The Lancet* Dec 21–28 (2): 1425.

Kantor, R. 2006. Impact of HIV-1 pol diversity on drug resistance and its clinical implications. *Current Opinion in Infectious Diseases* 19 (6) (Dec): 594–606.

Kantor, R., and D. Katzenstein. 2004. Drug resistance in non-subtype B HIV-1. *Journal of Clinical Virology: The Official Publication of the Pan American Society for Clinical Virology* 29 (3) (Mar): 152–9.

Katongole-Mbidde, E., C. Banura, and M. Nakakeeto. 1989. Diagnostic implications of genital Kaposi's sarcoma. *East African Medical Journal* 66 (8) (Aug): 499–502.

Kawuma, Annet. 2011. Coping to antiretroviral therapy: Strategies and modifying factors among adolescents at Mbarara regional referral hospital paediatric immune suppression syndrome clinic. MPH thesis, Mbarara University of Science & Technology.

Keller, Evelyn Fox. 1995. Gender and science: Origin, history and politics. *Osiris* 10: 27–38.

Kelly, Ann. 2011. Remember Bambali: Evidence, ethics and the co-production of truth. In *Evidence, ethos and experiment: The anthropology and history of medical research in Africa,* ed. Wenzel Geissler and Catherine Molyneux, 229–244. New York: Berghahn Books.

Kelly, Ann, and P. W. Geissler. 2011. The value of transnational medical research. *Journal of Cultural Economy* 4 (1): 3–10.

King, Nicholas B. 2002. Security, disease, commerce: Ideologies of postcolonial global health. *Social Studies of Science* 32 (5–6): 763–789.

Kinomoto, M., R. Appiah-Opong, J. A. Brandful, M. Yokoyama, N. Nii-Trebi, E. Ugly-Kwame, H. Sato, et al. 2005. HIV-1 proteases from drug-naive West African patients are differentially less susceptible to protease inhibitors. *Clinical Infectious Diseases: An Official Publication of the Infectious Diseases Society of America* 41 (2) (Jul 15): 243–51.

Knorr-Cetina, Karin. 1995. Laboratory studies: The cultural approach to the study of science. In *Handbook of science and technology studies,* ed. Sheila Jasanoff, Gerald Markle, James Petersen and Trevor Pinch, 140–166. Thousand Oaks: Sage Publications.

————. 1981. *The manufacture of knowledge: An essay on the constructivist and contextual nature of science*. New York: Pergamon Press.

Kohler, R. E. 1993. Drosophila: A life in the laboratory. *Journal of the History of Biology* 26 (2): 281–310.

Kolata, Gina. 2012. Bits of mystery DNA, far from 'junk,' play a crucial role. *New York Times*, September 6.

Koplan, J. P., T. C. Bond, M. H. Merson, K. S. Reddy, M. H. Rodriguez, N. K. Sewankambo, J. N. Wasserheit, and Consortium of Universities for Global Health Executive Board. 2009. Towards a common definition of global health. *Lancet* 373 (9679) (Jun 6): 1993–5.

Laeyendecker, O., X. Li, M. Arroyo, F. McCutchan, R. Gray, M. Wawer, and et al. 2006. The effect of HIV subtype on rapid disease progression in Rakai, Uganda. Paper presented at Conference on Retroviruses and Opportunistic Infections, Denver, CO. Abstract #44LB. Feb 6.

Lairumbi, Geoffrey, Michael Parker, Raymond Fitzpatrick, and Michael C. English. 2012. Forms of benefit sharing undertaken in global health research in resource poor settings: A qualitative study of stakeholders' views in Kenya. *Philosophy, Ethics, and Humanities in Medicine* 7 (7): 1–8.

Lakoff, Andrew. 2010. Two regimes of global health. *Humanity* 1 (1): 59–79.

Lakoff, Andrew, and Stephen J. Collier, ed. 2008. *Biosecurity interventions: Global health and security in question*. New York: Columbia University Press.

Lampland, M., and Susan Leigh Star, ed. 2009. *Standards and their stories: How quantifying, classifying, and normalizing practices shape everyday life*. Ithaca: Cornell University Press.

Landecker, Hannah. 2000. Immortality, in vitro: a history of the HeLa cell line. In *Biotechnology and culture: Bodies, anxieties, ethics*, ed. Paul Brodwin, 53–74. Bloomington: Indiana University Press.

Langwick, Stacey. 2011. *Bodies, politics, and African healing: The matter of maladies in Tanzania*. Bloomington: Indiana University Press.

Latour, Bruno. 1999. *Pandora's hope: Essays on the reality of science studies*. Cambridge: Harvard University Press.

————. 1987. *Science in action: How to follow scientists and engineers through society*. Cambridge: Harvard University Press.

————. 1983. Give me a laboratory and I will raise the world. In *Science observed: Perspectives on the social study of science*, ed. Karin Knorr-Cetina and Michael Mulkay, 141–169. London: Sage Publications.

Latour, Bruno, and Steve Woolgar. 1979. *Laboratory life: The construction of scientific facts*. Princeton: Princeton University Press.

Leigh Brown, A. J., S. D. Frost, W. C. Mathews, K. Dawson, N. S. Hellmann, E. S. Daar, D. D. Richman, and S. J. Little. 2003. Transmission fitness of drug-resistant human immunodeficiency virus and the prevalence of resistance in the antiretroviral-treated population. *The Journal of Infectious Diseases* 187 (4) (Feb 15): 683–6.

Leland, John. 1996. The end of AIDS? *Newsweek*, Dec 2.

Lerner, B. H., R. M. Gulick, and N. N. Dubler. 1998. Rethinking nonadherence: Historical perspectives on triple-drug therapy for HIV disease. *Annals of Internal Medicine* 129 (7) (Oct 1): 573–8.

Livingston, Julie. 2012. *Improvising medicine: An African oncology ward in an emerging epidemic.* Durham: Duke University Press.

——. 2005. *Debility and the moral imagination in Botswana.* Bloomington: Indiana University Press.

Lock, Margaret. 1995. *Encounters with aging: Mythologies of menopause in Japan and North America.* Berkeley: University of California Press.

Lock, Margaret, and Vinh-Kim Nguyen. 2010. *An anthropology of biomedicine.* Malden, MA: Wiley-Blackwell.

Loue, S., and D. Okello. 2000. Research bioethics in the Ugandan context II: Procedural and substantive reform. *The Journal of Law, Medicine & Ethics: A Journal of the American Society of Law, Medicine & Ethics* 28 (2) (Summer): 165–73.

Loue, S., D. Okello, and M. Kawuma. 1996. Research bioethics in the Ugandan context: A program summary. *The Journal of Law, Medicine & Ethics: A Journal of the American Society of Law, Medicine & Ethics* 24 (1) (Spring): 47–53.

Lowe, Celia. 2006. *Wild profusion: Biodiversity conservation in an Indonesian archipelago.* Princeton: Princeton University Press.

Löwy, Ilana. 2000. Trustworthy knowledge and desperate patients: Clinical tests for new drugs from cancer to AIDS. In *Living and working with the new medical technologies: Intersections of inquiry,* ed. Margaret Lock, Allen Young and Alberto Cambrosio, 49–81. Cambridge, UK: Cambridge University Press.

Luedke, Tracy, and Harry West, ed. 2006. *Borders and healers: Brokering therapeutic resources in southeast Africa.* Bloomington and Indianapolis: Indiana University Press.

Lynch, Michael. 1985. *Art and artifact in laboratory science: A study of shop work and shop talk in a research laboratory.* Studies in ethnomethodology. London, Boston: Routledge & Kegan Paul.

Macfarlane, S. B., M. Jacobs, and E. E. Kaaya. 2008. In the name of global health: Trends in academic institutions. *Journal of Public Health Policy* 29 (4) (Dec): 383–401.

Mahajan, Manjari. 2006. Right to certainty: AIDS activism in South Africa. Paper presented at the Annual Meeting of the Society for the Social Studies of Science, Vancouver, BC. November 1–5.

Malkki, Lisa. 1992. National geographic: The rooting of peoples and the territorialization of national identity among scholars and refugees. *Cultural Anthropology* 7 (2): 24–44.

Mamdani, Mahmood. 2011. The importance of research in a university. *Pambazuka News* 526: April 21. Accessed February 2, 2013, http://pambazuka.org/en/category/features/72782.

Marcus, George. 1998. *Ethnography through thick and thin.* Princeton: Princeton University Press.

Markowitz, M., H. Mohri, S. Mehandru, A. Shet, L. Berry, et al. 2005. Infection with multidrug resistant, dual-tropic HIV-1 and rapid progression to AIDS: A case report. *The Lancet* 365(9464): 1031–1038.

Martin, Emily. 1991. The egg and the sperm: How science has constructed a romance based on stereotypical male-female roles. *Signs* 16 (3): 485–501.

Martinez-Cajas, J. L., N. Pant-Pai, M. B. Klein, and M. A. Wainberg. 2008. Role of genetic diversity amongst HIV-1 non-B subtypes in drug resistance: A systematic review of virologic and biochemical evidence. *AIDS Reviews* 10 (4) (Oct–Dec): 212–23.

Matsiko, Charles Wycliffe, and Julie Kiwanuka. 2003. A review of human resource for health in Uganda. *Health Policy and Development* 1 (1): 15–20.

Mbembe, Achille. 2001. *On the postcolony*. Berkeley: University of California Press.

McCoy, D., G. Kembhavi, J. Patel, and A. Luintel. 2009. The Bill and Melinda Gates Foundation's grant-making programme for global health. *The Lancet* 373 (9675) (May 9): 1645–53.

McFadden, Robert. 1991. A drug-resistant TB results in 13 deaths in New York prisons. *New York Times*, Nov. 16.

McGreal, Chris. 2007. Chinese aid to Africa may do more harm than good, Benn warns. *Guardian*, Feb 8.

M'charek, Amade. 2005. *The human genome diversity project: An ethnography of scientific practice*. Cambridge: Cambridge University Press.

McNeil, Donald. 2012. Bill Gates donates $750 million to shore up disease-fighting fund. *New York Times*, January 27.

———. 2011a. Two studies show pills can prevent HIV infection. *New York Times*, July 14.

———. 2011b. Clinton aims for 'AIDS-free generation.' *New York Times*, November 9.

———. 2010. As the need grows, the money for AIDS runs far short. *New York Times*, May 9.

———. 2003. Africans outdo U.S. in following AIDS therapy. *New York Times* September 3.

———. 1998. South Africa's bitter pill for world's drug makers. *New York Times*, March 29.

McNeil, M. C. 2005. Introduction: Postcolonial technoscience (special issue). *Science as Culture* 14 (2): 105–22.

Merson, Michael. Testimony to the Congressional Global Health Caucus. *American Universities' Engagement in Global Health*, Hearing, September 16, 2009. Accessed September 6, 2012. Available at http://csis.org/event/american-universities-engagement -global-health.

Merson, Michael, and Kimberly Chapman Page. 2009. *The dramatic expansion of university engagement in global health: Implications for U.S. policy*. Washington, D.C.: Center for Strategic and International Studies.

Mika Marissa. 2009. Biopsies, bugs, and ice: Sample collection and exchange in Uganda, 1970–1971. Paper presented at The Africa Seminar, Johns Hopkins University. March 27.

Milford, Phil. 2011. Teva sued by GlaxoSmithKline, Pfizer venture over patent on HIV medicine. *Bloomberg.com*, August 8. Accessed February 2, 2013, http://www.bloomberg .com/news/2011-08-08/teva-sued-by-glaxosmithkline-pfizer-venture-over-hiv-medicine .html.

Mogensen, Hanne O. 2005. Finding a path through the health unit: Practical experience of Ugandan patients. *Medical Anthropology* (24): 209–36.

Montagnier, L. 2002. Historical essay: A history of HIV discovery. *Science* 298 (5599) (Nov 29): 1727–8.

Mudimbe, V. Y. 1988. *The invention of Africa: Gnosis, philosophy, and the order of knowledge*. Bloomington: Indiana University Press.

Müeller-Rockstroh, Babette. 2007. Ultrasound travels: The politics of a medical technology in Ghana and Tanzania. PhD diss., Universitaire Pers Maastricht.

Mugerwa, R., P. Kaleebu, P. Mugyenyi, E. Katongole-Mbidde, D.Hom, et al. 2002. First trial of the HIV-1 vaccine in Africa: Ugandan experience. *BMJ* 324 (January 24): 226–9.

Mugyenyi, Peter. 2008. *Genocide by denial: How profiteering from HIV/AIDS killed millions.* Kampala: Fountain Publishers.

Mukherjee, Siddhartha. 2000. Take your medicine: Why cheap AIDS drugs for Africa might be dangerous. *New Republic.* Jul 24.

Muñoz, N., F. X. Bosch, X. Castellsague, M. Diaz, S. de Sanjose, D. Hammouda, K. V. Shah, and C. J. Meijer. 2004. Against which human papillomavirus types shall we vaccinate and screen? The international perspective. *International Journal of Cancer.* 111 (2) (Aug 20): 278–85.

Museum of Contemporary Photography. Reininger, Alon. 2008. Accessed September 10, 2012, http://collections.mocp.org/detail.php?type=related&kv=7598&t=people.

Mwenda, Andrew. 2005. Africans on Africa: Debt. *BBC News,* July 7. Accessed February 2, 2013, http://news.bbc.co.uk/2/hi/africa/4657139.stm.

Nader, Laura. 1996. Introduction: Anthropological inquiry into boundaries, power, and knowledge. In *Naked science: Anthropological inquiry into boundaries, power, and knowledge,* ed. Laura Nader, 1–28. London: Routledge.

———. 1972. Up the anthropologist: Perspectives gained from studying up. In *Reinventing anthropology,* ed. Dell Hymes, 282–310. New York: Pantheon.

Nambuya, A., N. Sewankambo, J. Mugerwa, R. Goodgame, and S. Lucas. 1988. Tuberculous lymphadenitis associated with human immunodeficiency virus (HIV) in Uganda. *Journal of Clinical Pathology* 41 (1) (Jan): 93–6.

Navarro, Mireya. 1992. Gauging threat of recalcitrant TB patients. *New York Times,* April 14.

Nelkin, Dorothy. 1995. Science controversies: The dynamics of public disputes in the United States. In *Handbook of science and technology studies,* ed. Sheila Jasanoff, Gerald Markle, James Petersen and Trevor Pinch, 444–456. Thousand Oaks: Sage Publications.

Nguyen, Vinh-Kim. 2010. *The republic of therapy: Triage and sovereignty in West Africa's time of AIDS.* Durham: Duke University Press.

———. 2009. Government-by-exception: Enrollment and experimentality in mass HIV treatment programmes in Africa. *Social Theory and Health* 7 (3): 196–217.

———. 2005. Antiretroviral globalism, biopolitics, and therapeutic citizenship. In *Global assemblages,* ed. Aihwa Ong, Stephen J. Collier. Malden, MA: Blackwell Publishers.

Nguyen, Vinh-Kim, and Karine Peschard. 2003. Anthropology, inequality, and disease: A review. *Annual Review of Anthropology* (32): 447–64.

Nkengasong, J. N, C. Adje-Toure, and P. J. Weidle. 2004. HIV antiretroviral drug resistance in Africa. *AIDS Reviews* 6 (1) (Jan–Mar): 4–12.

Okeke, Iruka. 2011. *Divining without seeds: The case for strengthening laboratory medicine in Africa.* Ithaca: Cornell University Press.

Ong, Aihwa, and Stephen J. Collier, ed. 2005. *Global assemblages: Technology, politics and ethics as anthropological problems.* Malden, MA: Blackwell.

Oreskes, Naomi. 1997. Objectivity or heroism? On the invisibility of women in science. *Osiris* 11: 87–113.

Ortner, Sherry. 1995. Resistance and the problem of ethnographic refusal. *Comparative Studies in Society and History* 37 (1): 173–93.

Orzech, Kay, and Mark Nichter. 2008. From resilience to resistance: Political ecological lessons from antibiotic and pesticide resistance. *Annual Review of Anthropology* 37: 267–82.

Packard, R. M. 1989. *White plague, black labor: Tuberculosis and the political economy of health and disease in South Africa*. Berkeley: University of California Press.

Pargman, D, and J. Palme. 2009. ASCII imperialism. In *Standards and their stories: How quantifying, classifying, and normalizing practices shape everyday life,* ed. M. Lampland and Susan Leigh Star. Ithaca: Cornell University Press.

Parker, R. 2002. The global HIV/AIDS pandemic, structural inequalities, and the politics of international health. *American Journal of Public Health* 92 (3) (Mar): 343–6.

Paterson, D. L., S. Swindells, J. Mohr, M. Brester, E. N. Vergis, et al. 2000. Adherence to protease inhibitor therapy and outcomes in patients with HIV infection. *Annals of Internal Medicine* 133 (1) (Jul 4): 21–30.

Paulson, Tom. 2008. Global health seen as big business for Seattle. *Seattle Post-Intelligencer,* October 23.

Perez-Pena, Richard. 2005. Chilled by findings, investigators dreaded the mounting evidence. *New York Times,* February 12.

Petryna, Adriana. 2009. *When experiments travel: Clinical trials and the global search for human subjects*. Princeton: Princeton University Press.

Pfeiffer, J. 2002. African independent churches in Mozambique: Healing the afflictions of inequality. *Medical Anthropology Quarterly* 16 (2): 176–99.

Pfeiffer, J., and R. Chapman. 2010. Anthropological perspectives on structural adjustment and public health. *Annual Review of Anthropology* 39: 149–65.

Pfeiffer, J., M. Nichter, and Critical Anthropology of Global Health Special Interest Group. 2008. What can critical medical anthropology contribute to global health? A health systems perspective. *Medical Anthropology Quarterly* 22 (4) (Dec): 410–5.

PhRMA (Pharmaceutical Research and Manufacturers of America). 2006. Danger ahead: Drug resistant strains shows there are no simple solutions. Accessed July 29, 2008, http://web.archive.org/web/20061009203949/http://world.phrma.org/challenges .drug.resistance.html.html.

Piller, Charles. 2005. AIDS experts awaken to a false alarm. *Los Angeles Times*. June 5.

Pigg, Stacy Leigh. 2001. Languages of sex and AIDS in Nepal: Notes on the social production of commensurability. *Cultural Anthropology* 16 (4): 481–541.

Popp, D., and J. D. Fisher. 2002. First, do no harm: A call for emphasizing adherence and HIV prevention interventions in active antiretroviral therapy programs in the developing world. *AIDS (London, England)* 16 (4) (Mar 8): 676–8.

Powell, Alvin. 2010. Panel examines New England's strategic contributions, role in global health. *Harvard Gazette,* April 27.

Puget Sound Regional Council. 2012. Global health. Accessed September 1, 2012, http://psrc.org/econdev/global-health/.

Rainey, Lisa. 2006. Who discovered HIV: Gallo, Montagnier or both? *Dallas Voice,* July 7.

Reardon, Jenny. 2005. *Race to the finish: Identity and governance in an age of genomics.* Princeton: Princeton University Press.

Redfield, Peter. 2005. Doctors, borders, and life in crisis. *Cultural Anthropology* 20 (3): 328–61.

Redfield, Peter, and Erica Bornstein. 2010. An introduction to the anthropology of humanitarianism. In *Forces of compassion: Humanitarianism between ethics and politics,* ed. Peter Redfield and Erica Bornstein, 3–30. Santa Fe: School for Advanced Research Press.

Revuluri, Sindhumathi. 2007. On anxiety and absorption: Musical encounters with the exotique in fin-de-siècle France. PhD diss., Princeton University.

Rheinberger, Hans-Jorg, and Jean-Paul Gaudilliere. 2004. Introduction. In *Classical genetics research and its legacy: The mapping cultures of 20th century genetics,* ed. Hans-Jorg Rheinberger and Jean-Paul Gaudilliere, 1–7. New York: Routledge.

Richman, D. D., S. C. Morton, T. Wrin, N. Hellmann, S. Berry, M. F. Shapiro, and S. A. Bozzette. 2004. The prevalence of antiretroviral drug resistance in the United States. *AIDS (London, England)* 18 (10) (Jul 2): 1393–401.

Rose, Nikolas. 2007. *The politics of life itself: Biomedicine, power, and subjectivity in the twenty-first century.* Princeton: Princeton University Press.

———. 2001. The politics of life itself. *Theory, Culture and Society* 18 (6): 1–30.

Rottenburg, Richard. 2009. Social and public experiments and new figurations of science and politics in postcolonial Africa. *Postcolonial Studies* 12 (4): 423–40.

Rushton, Simon, and Owain David Williams. 2011. Private actors in global health governance. In *Partnerships and foundations in global health governance,* ed. Simon Rushton and Owain David Williams, 1–28. London: Palgrave Macmillan.

Sahoo, Sananda. 2010. U.S. AIDS funding flat-lining, groups complain. *Inter Press Service News Agency,* March 12.

Santora, Mark, and Lawrence Altman. 2005. Rare and aggressive HIV reported in New York. *New York Times,* February 12.

Schoenfeld, D. A., D. M. Finkelstein, and D. D. Richman. 1993. Designing phase II studies of chemotherapy for HIV infection using CD4 as an end-point. *AIDS (London, England)* 7 (7) (Jul): 955–8.

Schoepf, B. 2003. Uganda: Lessons for AIDS control in Africa. *Review of African Political Economy* 30 (98): 553–72.

Seattle Center Foundation. 2011. The next fifty: A six-month dialogue about our future. Accessed September 1, 2012, http://www.thenextfifty.org/the-next-fifty/.

Senak, M. 1997. Predicting antiviral compliance: Physicians' responsibilities vs. patients' rights. *Journal of the International Association of Physicians in AIDS Care* 3 (6) (Jun): 45–8.

Sendagire, H., P. J. Easterbrook, I. Nankya, E. Arts, D. Thomas, and S. J. Reynolds. 2009. The challenge of HIV-1 antiretroviral resistance in Africa in the era of HAART. *AIDS Reviews* 11 (2) (Apr–Jun): 59–70.

Serwadda, D., R. D. Mugerwa, N. K. Sewankambo, A. Lwegaba, J. W. Carswell, G. B. Kirya, et al. 1985. Slim disease: A new disease in Uganda and its association with HTLV-III infection. *The Lancet* 2 (8460) (Oct 19): 849–52.

Seth, Suman. 2009. Putting knowledge in its place: Science, colonialism, and the postcolonial. *Postcolonial Studies* 12 (4): 373–88.

Sewankambo, N. K., R. D. Mugerwa, R. Goodgame, J. W. Carswell, A. Moody, et al. 1987a. Enteropathic AIDS in Uganda: An endoscopic, histological and microbiological study. *AIDS (London, England)* 1 (1) (May): 9–13.

Sewankambo, N. K., J. W. Carswell, R. D. Mugerwa, G. Lloyd, P. Kataaha, R. G. Downing, and S. Lucas. 1987b. HIV infection through normal heterosexual contact in Uganda. *AIDS (London, England)* 1 (2) (Jul): 113–6.

Shapin, Steven. 1989. The invisible technician. *American Scientist* 77 (Nov–Dec): 554–63.

Shapin, Steven, and Simon Schaffer. 1987. *Leviathan and the air pump: Hobbes, Boyle, and the experimental life.* Princeton: Princeton University Press.

Sheppard, H. W., M. S. Ascher, W. Winkelstein, E. Vittinghoff, D. Osmond, A. R. Moss, and S. Shiboski. 1993. Use of T lymphocyte subset analysis in the case definition for AIDS. *Journal of Acquired Immune Deficiency Syndromes* 6 (3) (Mar): 287–94.

Skloot, Rebecca. 2010. *The immortal life of Henrietta Lacks.* New York: Crown Publishers.

Smith, S. M. 2005. New York City HIV superbug: Fear or fear not? Retrovirology 2:14.

Sollitto, S., M. Mehlman, S. Youngner, and M. M. Lederman. 2001. Should physicians withhold highly active antiretroviral therapies from HIV-AIDS patients who are thought to be poorly adherent to treatment? *AIDS (London, England)* 15 (2) (Jan 26): 153–9.

Sontag, Deborah, and Lynda Richardson. 1997. Doctors withhold H.I.V. pill regimen from some. *New York Times,* March 2.

Sparke, Matthew. 2013. Health. In *The handbook of progress in human geography,* ed. Roger Lee, Noel Castree, Rob Kitchin, Vicky Lawson, Anssi Paasi, et al. Thousand Oaks: Sage Publications.

———. 2011. Global geographies. In *Seattle geographies,* ed. Michael Brown and Richard Morrill, 48–70. Seattle: University of Washington Press.

———. 1998. A map that roared and an original atlas: Canada, cartography and the narration of nation. *Annals of the Association of American Geographers* 88 (3): 464–95.

Specter, Michael. 2007. Darwin's surprise. *The New Yorker* (Dec 3): 64–73.

———. 1992. Neglected for years, TB is back with strains that are deadlier. *New York Times,* A1.

Spira, S., M. A. Wainberg, H. Loemba, D. Turner, and B. G. Brenner. 2003. Impact of clade diversity on HIV-1 virulence, antiretroviral drug sensitivity and drug resistance. *The Journal of Antimicrobial Chemotherapy* 51 (2) (Feb): 229–40.

Starr, Paul. 1982. *The social transformation of American medicine.* New York: Basic Books.

Stevens, W., S. Kaye, and T. Corrah. 2004. Antiretroviral therapy in Africa. *BMJ (Clinical Research Ed.)* 328 (7434) (Jan 31): 280–2.

Stewart, K., and N. Sewankambo. 2010. *Okukkera ng'omuzugu* (lost in translation): Understanding the social value of global health research for HIV/AIDS participants in Uganda. *Global Public Health* 5 (2): 164–80.

Stine, Gerald. 2004. *AIDS update.* Englewood Cliffs, NJ: Prentice Hall.

Sullivan, Andrew. 2001. Profit of doom? *New Republic,* Mar 26.

Sunder Rajan, Kauchik. 2006. *Biocapital: The constitution of post-genomic life.* Durham: Duke University Press.

Tang, J. W., and D. Pillay. 2004. Transmission of HIV-1 drug resistance. *Journal of Clinical Virology* 30 (1): 1–10.

Taylor, B. S., M. E. Sobieszczky, F. E. McCutchan, and S. M. Hammer. 2008. The challenge of HIV-1 subtype diversity. *The New England Journal of Medicine* 359 (18) (Oct 30): 1965–6.

Tchetgen, E., E. H. Kaplan, and G. H. Friedland. 2001. Public health consequences of screening patients for adherence to highly active antiretroviral therapy. *Journal of Acquired Immune Deficiency Syndromes (1999)* 26 (2) (Feb 1): 118–29.

Thomas, Lynn. 2003. *The politics of the womb: Women, reproduction, and the state in Kenya.* Berkeley: University of California Press.

Thompson, M. A., J. A. Aberg, P. Cahn, J. S. Montaner, G. Rizzardini, et al. 2010. Antiretroviral treatment of adult HIV infection: 2010 recommendations of the international AIDS society-USA panel. *JAMA: The Journal of the American Medical Association* 304 (3) (Jul 21): 321–33.

Thomson, M. M., and R. Najera. 2001. Travel and the introduction of human immunodeficiency virus type 1 non-B subtype genetic forms into western countries. *Clinical Infectious Diseases: An Official Publication of the Infectious Diseases Society of America* 32 (12) (Jun 15): 1732–7.

Thornton, Robert J. 2008. *Unimagined community: Sex, networks, and AIDS in Uganda and South Africa.* Berkeley: University of California Press.

Ticktin, Miriam. 2006. Where ethics and politics meet: The violence of humanitarianism in France. *American Ethnologist* 33 (1): 33–49.

Tilley, Helen. 2011. *Africa as a living laboratory: Empire, development, and the problem of scientific knowledge.* Chicago: University of Chicago Press.

Treichler, Paula. 1987. AIDS, homophobia, and biomedical discourse: An epidemic of signification. *October* 43 (Winter): 263–305.

Tsing, Anna. 2005. *Friction: An ethnography of global connection.* Princeton: Princeton University Press.

Turnbull, David. 2004. Genetic mapping: Approaches to the spatial topography of genetics. In *Classical genetics research and its legacy: The mapping cultures of 20th century genetics,* ed. Hans-Jorg Rheinberger and Jean-Paul Gaudilliere, 207–219. New York: Routledge.

———. 1989. *Maps are territories, science is an atlas.* Chicago: University of Chicago Press.

UCSF Global Health Sciences. 2012. Education and training: Curriculum. Accessed September 8, 2012. Available from http://globalhealthsciences.ucsf.edu/education -training/clinical-scholars/curriculum.

UNAIDS, and WHO. 2006. *AIDS epidemic update: Special report on HIV/AIDS— December 2006.* Geneva: United Nations Programme on AIDS (UNAIDS).

UNDP (United Nations Development Programme). 2010. *The real wealth of nations: Pathways to human development.* Accessed February 2, 2013, http://hdr.undp.org/en /reports/global/hdr2010/.

UNICEF. 2006. *Pneumonia: The forgotten killer of children.* UNICEF/WHO. Accessed February 2, 2012, http://www.unicef.org/publications/index_35626.html.

University of Minnesota Medical School. 2010. International medical research and education program. Accessed May 11, 2010, http://web.archive.org/web/20100610204252 /http://www.meded.umn.edu/imer/.

University of Washington. 2007. *Phase I global support project focus group report, January 12.* Accessed February 2, 2013, http://f2.washington.edu/fm/globalsupport/about -global-support-project.

Vaughan, Meghan. 1991. *Curing their ills: Colonial power and African illness.* Stanford: Stanford University Press.

Villareal, Luis P. 2004. Are viruses alive? *Scientific American,* December: 96–102.

Volberding, P. A. 2005. The New York case: Lessons being learned. *Annals of Internal Medicine* 142(10): 866–868.

Wainberg, M. A., and B. G. Brenner. 2012. The impact of HIV genetic polymorphisms and subtype differences on the occurrence of resistance to antiretroviral drugs. *Molecular Biology International* 2012: 256982.

Waldholz, Michael. 1996. Precious pills: New AIDS treatment raises tough questions of who will get it. *Wall Street Journal,* July 3.

Walensky, R. P., A. D. Paltiel, E. Losina, L. M. Mercincavage, B. R. Schackman, et al. 2006. The survival benefits of AIDS treatment in the United States. *The Journal of Infectious Diseases* 194 (1) (Jul 1): 11–9.

Watson-Verran, Helen, and David Turnbull. 1995. Science and other indigenous knowledge systems. In *Handbook of science and technology studies,* ed. Sheila Jasanoff, Gerald Markle, Trevor Pinch and James Petersen, 115–139. Thousand Oaks: Sage Publications.

Watts, J. M., K. K. Dang, R. J. Gorelick, C. W. Leonard, J. W. Bess, et al. 2009. Architecture and secondary structure of an entire HIV-1 RNA genome. *Nature* 460 (7256) (Aug 6): 711–6.

Weidle, P. J., R. Downing, C. Sozi, R. Mwebaze, G. Rukundo, et al. 2003. Development of phenotypic and genotypic resistance to antiretroviral therapy in the UN-AIDS HIV drug access initiative—Uganda. *AIDS (London, England)* 17 Suppl 3 (Jul): S39–48.

Weidle, P. J., N. Wamai, P. Solberg, C. Liechty, S. Sendagala, et al. 2006. Adherence to antiretroviral therapy in a home-based AIDS care programme in rural Uganda. *The Lancet* 368 (9547) (Nov 4): 1587–94.

Weiser, S. D., D. M. Tuller, E. A. Frongillo, J. Senkungu, N. Mukiibi, and D. R. Bangsberg. 2010. Food insecurity and a barrier to sustained antiretroviral adherence in Uganda. *PLoS One* 5(4)(Apr 28): e10340.

Wendland, Claire. 2012. Moral maps and medical imaginaries: Clinical tourism at Malawi's college of medicine. *American Anthropologist* 114 (1): 108–22.

———. 2010. *A heart for the work: Journeys through an African medical school.* Chicago: University of Chicago Press.

———. 2008. Research, therapy, and bioethical hegemony: The controversy over perinatal AZT trials in Africa. *African Studies Review* 51 (3): 1–23.

Westerhaus, Michael, and Arachu Castro. 2006. How do intellectual property law and international trade agreements affect access to antiretroviral therapy? *PLoS Medicine* 3, (8), doi:10.1371/journal.pmed.0030332.

WHO (World Health Organization). HIV drug resistance fact sheet, April 2011. Accessed June 12, 2012, http://www.who.int/hiv/facts/drug_resistance/en/index .html.

WHO, UNICEF, and UNAIDS. 2011. *Global HIV/AIDS response: Epidemic update and health sector progress towards universal access: Progress report 2011.* Geneva: World Health Organization.

Whyte, S. R. 2011. Writing knowledge and acknowledgment: Possibilities in medical research. In *Evidence, ethos, and experiment: The anthropology and history of medical research in Africa,* ed. P. W. Geissler and Catherine Molyneux, 29–56. New York: Berghahn Books.

———. Pharmaceuticals as folk medicine: Transformations in the social relations of health care in Uganda. *Culture, Medicine, and Psychiatry* 16: 163–86.

———. 1991. Medicines and self-help: The privatization of health care in eastern Uganda. In *Changing Uganda: The dilemmas of structural adjustment and revolutionary change,* ed. H. B. Hansen and M. Twaddle, 130–148. London: James Currey.

Whyte, S. R., M. A. Whyte, L. Meinert and B. Kyaddondo. 2004. Treating AIDS: Dilemmas of unequal access in Uganda. *Journal of Social Aspects of HIV/AIDS Research Alliance* 1 (1): 14–26.

Wilson, Phill, Kai Wright, and Michael T. Isbell. 2008. *Left behind: Black America, A neglected priority in the global AIDS epidemic.* Los Angeles: Black AIDS Institute.

Winner, Langdon. 1980. Do artifacts have politics? *Daedalus* 109 (1): 121–136.

World Bank. 1999. *Confronting AIDS: Public priorities in a global epidemic.* Revised edition. Oxford University Press for the World Bank.

INDEX